STRESS

STRESS

HOW TO DE-STRESS
WITHOUT DOING LESS

Dr Kate Middleton

LION

Copyright © 2009 Kate Middleton
This edition copyright © 2009 Lion Hudson

The author asserts the moral right
to be identified as the author of this work

A Lion Book
an imprint of
Lion Hudson plc
Wilkinson House, Jordan Hill Road,
Oxford OX2 8DR, England
www.lionhudson.com

ISBN 978 0 7459 5373 1 (UK)
ISBN 978 0 8254 7919 9 (US)

Distributed by:
UK: Marston Book Services, PO Box 269, Abingdon, Oxon OX14 4YN
USA: Trafalgar Square Publishing, 814 N. Franklin Street, Chicago, IL 60610
USA Christian Market: Kregel Publications, PO Box 2607, Grand Rapids,
MI 49501

First edition 2009

10 9 8 7 6 5 4 3 2 1 0

This book has been printed on paper and board independently certified
as having been produced from sustainable forests.

A catalogue record for this book is available
from the British Library

Typeset in 10.5/14 Baskerville BT

Printed and bound in Great Britain by CPI Cox & Wyman, Reading.

Contents

Introduction

In my job I work with all kinds of different people, in lots of different situations – in their workplace, in schools, in the community, at work and at home. As I share in people's lives, I come across a variety of issues. Listening to them as they talk about their journeys, the things they have been through and the difficulties they are struggling with, has given me the opportunity and the privilege of sharing in many people's experiences of what their own emotions can lead them to. I have learned a lot – far more than I ever learned in any of my years of formal studying – about what the things life throws at normal people can push them to: the extremes of emotions, difficulties with addictions, traumatic memories, and difficult and unhelpful beliefs about themselves and the world around them.

Writing this book has given me another opportunity to share some of the insights I have gained in my work. But if I am honest, writing *this* book has been very different for one key reason. Although I understand them very well, on the whole the issues I have covered in my previous books have been things that I do not struggle with myself. They are things I have learned about through sharing the experiences of others, through witnessing their struggles and applying the theory and fact that I already knew. This issue, however, is one that I readily confess I face day to day, like so many other people – and no doubt like you, seeing as you are reading this book.

Stress is a modern-day plague, something that very few of us escape – something that we probably all have to think about as it follows us every day. Stress is always there in the background, lurking behind us, following throughout our lives and ready to hit at moments we least expect it. Stress can take many forms and come from many sources. Like a lot of people, I am someone who likes to fill life with many different things. I like to achieve things, to accomplish things, to fit plenty into my days. Too easily I see things that need doing and take on the responsibility of doing them! But my own experience, starting with life as a medical student years ago, has taught me (though I have not been quick to learn it!) that if I do want to push myself that hard and achieve the things I aim for, I must not forget to make sure I handle stress well.

Stress can often be an unwanted companion along the road of life. We may not like it but it's there! Too many people I have worked with have had months or years stolen by stress, or are facing the risk that they might have to give up things they love or stifle something of the person they are, because stress is having too serious an impact on them. We have to be sensible where stress is concerned. Finding the balance of how much we really can squeeze into life means we have to learn how to fight stress in the best way possible.

This book is about how to deal with stress – how to reduce it where we can and live with it when we can't (we may as well accept it is unlikely to vanish completely). It is about how to stop stress from taking over our lives and ultimately taking bits of our lives from us. So join me on a lifelong journey of fighting this battle – negotiating with stress and trying to come out as the winner!

PART 1

Understanding stress

WHAT IS STRESS AND HOW MIGHT IT AFFECT YOU?

1 Why worry about stress?

Stress, it seems, is everywhere! In fact, in my job, if there is one thing that ordinary people ask me about more than any other – people of all ages, from all walks of life, people working, people bringing up children, people with worries for themselves and people who are worried about others – it's stress! It doesn't take long if you are reading the daily papers, scanning the news channels or reading reports on the internet to find something referring to stress – something that has triggered stress, the impact stress has on a situation or on certain people, the medical or psychological impact of stress... Stress has become something that almost everyone seems to be concerned about, yet, at the same time, something that we all feel we are at the mercy of. If you get a group of friends together to chat about how their life is going, it won't be long before stress comes up. Stress is a key issue in the workplace, where managers are expected to think about how the jobs they give people impact on them in terms of stress. It is discussed at schools, where teachers now often find they need to introduce programmes designed to help pupils cope with stress, as well as teaching them the usual subjects. Even very young children are not immune, with recent findings that even pre-school children can be affected by stress, leading some nursery schools to introduce yoga and relaxation classes for toddlers. As one mum said to me recently, 'How stressed can you be by four years old?'

So, just how big an issue is 'stress'?

Are media reports highlighting a genuine problem, or are we just making too big a deal out of something that decades ago people would just have got on with? Are stress levels really rising, and how should we be responding to the apparent tidal wave of related problems? Concerns over rising stress levels in the UK have even led to warnings from politicians of a 'epidemic of mental distress'. Should we be concerned?

There is certainly plenty of evidence showing apparent problems linked to or caused by stress. Research shows that one in three adults feels stressed every day, with younger adults feeling the pressure most – around half of people in their early twenties say that they feel under pressure most days. Stress has been linked to all kinds of physical problems including heart disease, problems with skin conditions such as eczema, and sleep problems. One study even found that women working in stressful jobs were more likely to start the menopause earlier than their more chilled-out colleagues.

Stress has also been linked to problems with mental health and emotional illnesses such as anxiety and depression. One study looking at a group of people in their early thirties found that work stress was related to the start of problems with depression and anxiety in 45 per cent of cases. The people studied worked in a wide variety of professions, but all reported stresses such as long hours, lack of control over their work and tight deadlines. About one person in four develops a new problem with anxiety or depression in any given year, but it seems the risk is doubled if you work in a high-pressure job.

Stress in the workplace is one of the big issues that we see discussed in the press. The reason for this is clear. Government statistics in the UK say that around one in five workers say they feel extremely stressed while at work, with about 14 per cent saying that they feel their work stress is making them ill. This equates to around 5 million people who are unwell as a result of work stress. Work-related stress accounted for an estimated 13.5 million lost working days in Britain in one year alone (2007–2008). The same trend is seen in other countries. In Australia stress costs more to the economy than any other illness, and figures from the US suggest that around $300 billion ($7,500 per employee) is spent every year on stress-related issues. This cost comes from compensation claims, absenteeism and lost productivity, because even when people are at work, stress can seriously affect the work that they do – or don't do. The term 'presenteeism' describes those who are at work but are not working effectively because of stress. We've all had days like that, where you feel as if you have run around all day like a headless chicken but actually accomplished next to nothing! One study reports that on average, Australian adults lose six working days every year through presenteeism. Meanwhile, workers across the world are working longer hours and feeling under more pressure than in previous decades. A report looking at workers from thirty different countries found that one fifth of those workers report feeling very high levels of stress.

The impact of this stress is not something to take lightly. One study following a group of civil servants over a period of 12 years found those who reported that their job was stressful were 70 per cent more likely to develop heart disease than those who were stress-free. In fact, three quarters of executives admit that their stress adversely affects not just their work performance but also their home life and relationships. 65 per cent of Americans admit they lose sleep every night due to stress, and depression linked to stress is predicted to be the number one occupational illness of the twenty-first century. These are statistics and reports that are really worrying if you take the time to think about them, especially as many of us, if we're honest, live lives where stress is a daily reality, not just at work but throughout our lives as we juggle many different responsibilities. For example, mothers seem to be at particular risk, especially those who balance work with looking after young children. Research reports that globally one in four mothers who work full-time as well as look after children report feeling stressed every day.

Young people and stress

It isn't just adults who are struggling with stress. Stress seems to be an issue right from the start of childhood. Some experts claim that growing up in the UK places far too much pressure on children – pressure that is suggested to be behind the growing numbers of emotional and mental health problems such as eating disorders, self harm, serious depression and even suicidal behaviour among increasingly young children and teens. Those working within schools report clearly the impact that testing and exams can have on even very young children (the first formal tests – SATS – starting at just seven years old). Problems with exam stress in school children have led to special campaigns from charities such as ChildLine, and many bodies are concerned about the effect that exam worries have on young children. Although government ministers in the UK have been quick to point out that SATS at this age are not formal exams, many teachers and parents are concerned about the obvious anxiety and stress that they produce in children, particularly those who are vulnerable or who may be 'coached' or pushed by anxious parents or teachers concerned about league tables.

Of course, it isn't just exams that cause young people stress. Current culture means that teenagers in particular report feeling under pressure from many different perspectives, including romantic relationships and sex, issues such as drinking alcohol and taking drugs, family pressure and family breakdown, health worries and concerns over their future. Growing up seems to have become a barrage of one stress after another, and it seems that many young people are struggling to cope. Helping children to understand stress and the impact it has on us is becoming a vital part of parenting today, but with many parents themselves struggling under the weight of stress, few feel equipped to help teach their children how to cope. In fact, research suggests that if parents are themselves stressed, it has a direct impact on children who may be more prone to infections and illness as well as struggling to know how to cope with stress and anxiety themselves.

Non-work sources of stress

Meanwhile, for the adults, it isn't just work that is stressing us out. One study found that more than half of us admit that we are kept awake at night by worries about health risks and financial problems or concerns about world events such as climate change and terrorism. All this stress means that only

3 per cent of adults get the recommended amount of sleep. Changes to lifestyle, with us all tending to do less exercise and eat less healthily, have also had an impact on the way that stress affects us. Many adults admit that they feel they are simply not operating at their best because of the effect that stress has on them day to day. Stress seems to make us struggle with planning and organization, affect simple things such as memory and communication, and generally make our lives more difficult. In fact, among the various reports of how stress affects our health are some that seem to suggest it really does have an impact on how well our brains work, with research indicating that severe stress can even cause cells to die within the brain, affecting functions such as learning and memory.

All in all, reports about stress are enough to make you want to retire to a desert island in search of the ultimate stress-free ideal. Indeed, many people do that every year as they jet off on their holidays in search of a stress-free pocket of time in the middle of their stress-filled lives – though they might do well to read the research that places holidays among the most stressful experiences we can have in day-to-day life! As we work longer and longer hours, the 'work hard, play hard' culture designed to help us cope with stress may actually be causing as many problems as it solves, with people struggling with exhaustion and resorting to alcohol and drugs in order to help them wind down and chase that stress-free idyll. Those in stressful and pressured professions are at an increased risk of struggling with problems such as addictions, and worries about the amount young professionals are drinking in particular are growing among health professionals and government ministers alike.

Why is stress such an important issue?

So, what is the most important message behind all the stories, claims and disputed 'facts' that are reported about stress? Whatever the specific details are, stress seems to stop us from being able to operate at our best. And here is one fact that is not debated. Whereas mild stress can actually make us work better, someone placed under severe stress will not be able to work as well, as efficiently or as productively as someone who is not. Put simply, this kind of chronic, intense stress is at risk of stopping us from reaching our full potential. Much as we worry about the academic qualifications that children and young people achieve, the reality in our culture today is that how well they do in their chosen field of work may well be determined not by their ability but by how well they deal with stress. This means that in some working environments or schools, where people are, by definition, selected on the basis that they are highly able and clever, who enjoys the most success in the long term may well be predicted by looking at how those people respond to stressful situations and how well they cope with that stress.

Whether we like it or not, stress is a reality and, for most of us, something that we will have to learn to deal with. So, what can we do? Too often the response to someone struggling with stress is about how they can get out of that stressful environment, how they can remove or reduce sources of stress. But for many of us, our lifestyles and/or work produce sources of stress that are not optional. It is no good telling a stressed-out parent to stop spending so much time with their children! And for others, although they could stop doing the things that are causing them stress, that would mean giving up things that they actually love – things that make them who they are supposed to be. If we take someone

17

whose dream has always been to be a lawyer, and tell them that they need to give this job up because stress is making them ill, we take away from them part of who they are. We need to be sensible. Stress management may well mean making some changes to our lives. But we also need to find solutions for stress that don't just involve having to do a lot less. In the end, stress management is not about doing less; it is about learning how to cope better with the stress that is involved with being who we are, having the responsibilities that we have, and doing the kinds of things we like to do. So, if we want to be able to carry on pushing ourselves hard and keep getting the most we can out of life, we need to understand stress and be really good at dealing with it. That, in a nutshell, is what this book is about.

2 What is stress?

So, before we get too much further, let's look at what exactly we mean by 'stress'. Most people think they have a pretty good idea of what stress is. Stress is something often talked about, mentioned in media reports and linked with all kinds of issues. The word is one we come across all the time, but it's important to be really clear exactly what it is – and of what I mean when I use the word in this book. This is because one of the most important things to understand about stress is that the way a lot of people use the word often reveals a basic misunderstanding about what stress is. Often when I start working with someone who is struggling with stress-related problems, what they mean by the word 'stress' is often not the same as I do.

So who gets 'stressed'?

Think about it. When 'stress' is talked about, the word is generally used to describe something emotional – something going on in our minds – or stress is blamed for something that happened which we wish had not happened. So, if someone is not coping very well with something demanding – be it a job, small child or life crisis – we talk about them being 'stressed'. When that colleague goes off sick again and again with something that just won't get better, we might hear someone saying that it is because he or she lets themselves get so 'stressed'. Or, if someone is suddenly very moody, seeming grumpy and unreasonable, or, at the other extreme, prone to taking things too personally and bursting into tears all the time, very often people will put it down to 'stress'. This use of the word 'stress' perhaps strongly shows its origin – in the word 'distress'; originally stress described an emotional response. Even now dictionary definitions still show this tendency.[1]

What is also apparent in the way we talk about stress is a hint of the opinions we often have about it. Many of us talk about stress as though it were something we should ideally be able to avoid. We sometimes even look down on people who struggle with 'stress'. Very often people I work with are reluctant to admit that stress has anything to do with their problems and see it almost as admitting some kind of weakness. In high-flying and very demanding careers, where stress-related illness is common, it is often simply not done to admit that you find it difficult to deal with the stress. Managing to continue working under extreme stress can be seen as some kind of extra qualification or ability, as essential and valued as academic brilliance, and anyone who falters under the weight of that stress 'can't take the heat' or 'isn't up to it'.

In fact, if we're honest, most of us have a tendency to look down on someone who is showing too many signs of 'stress'. It's something that people do where any kind of emotional or 'mental health' problem is concerned. Most people like to think that the world is made up of two kinds of people – those who struggle with 'mental health' problems (including those who might struggle with 'stress') and those who don't. It's as if we can divide everyone we know into two categories. On the one hand are most of the people we know – in the 'happy and healthy' category. They are what we might call 'normal' and don't suffer from any emotional or mental health problems. They are happy and successful. Meanwhile, a few people we know would fall into the other category – the 'unhappy' or 'ill' box. These are the people who suffer from emotional or psychological ill health that has been significant enough to cause them to seek some kind of help. This is not generally thought to be a box you can move out of – once someone has had a mental health problem on the whole they are thought of as someone with that inherent 'weakness'. One friend of mine, who has been recovered for more than a decade from the serious psychological problems he developed in his early twenties, remembers the response he received when telling a friend about how he had been struggling to cope with recent pressures at work: 'Ah, but you have always been a bit "vulnerable", haven't you?'

Some people who are in the 'ill' category have struggled for a long time – often since their teens or early adult life. This leads to the conclusion that emotional and psychological problems are things that affect only a small proportion of people, who are in some way different or vulnerable. Every once in a while someone develops a problem in adult life for the first time, and this apparent change of category can take us by surprise. One person I worked with told me of the day she admitted at work that her long absence was not in fact due to a bad dose of flu but because she had been struggling with depression. She overheard two colleagues talking about her later on. 'I never knew she had those kind of problems,' one said to the other. 'It just goes to show you never can tell, can you?'

We like to believe in this 'either healthy or ill' system because it protects us from a very basic truth. It means that if, so far, we have not had any emotional problems, we fool ourselves into thinking that we probably never will. In fact, most so-called 'mental health' problems can and often do affect anyone, including those people you might think least likely to suffer; those people who have never suffered from anything before. My job brings me into contact every day with people who are perfectly 'normal' but who have encountered difficult or extreme experiences in life and as a result found themselves struggling with some kind of emotional problem. The truth is that, in some ways, there is nothing more scary than the kinds of things that 'normal' people like you and me can be pushed to if life throws things at us that are beyond our capacity to cope with.

Stress is linked to the development of almost all mental health problems and, as we will see, can trigger both physical and psychological ill health. But in the same way that we like to believe we are not at risk of mental health problems, we also often think we are immune from the impact of stress. Particularly in a culture where life is jam-packed, full of pressure and the need to achieve, we feel that we should manage to be superhuman and cope with all the things thrown at us. We'll freely admit that life is 'stressful' but put ourselves under pressure never to show any signs of that stress. We slip into believing that by ignoring stress we can avoid it having any impact on us.

So, what is the truth about stress?

If you listen to a doctor or psychologist talking about stress, you'll quickly realize that they mean something much more than a response that is all in our minds. In fact, stress is a very real physical phenomenon that causes real physiological changes within our bodies *and* our brains. Stress is something that we all need to be aware of, because many of the signs and symptoms stress can trigger are actually caused by the physiological changes that it has triggered.

This doesn't mean that the way we respond – emotionally and psychologically – to situations, or indeed to stress, doesn't have an impact. Our individual response to difficult things, as well as some basic things about the way our minds work, can certainly make stress more or less of a problem, and we'll talk about some of these things in later chapters. But at the root of stress are real physical changes with real physical impacts.

What we call stress refers to a response that our brain triggers when the situation we find ourselves in requires us to do something specific or be ready to react in a certain way. It might be that something is happening now, or that our brain has detected a chance that something might happen and so primes our body to be alert in case it does. The actual response could be any number of things. It may be about getting us physically ready, such as the well-known 'fight or flight' response that occurs if we feel threatened or at risk. Or stress can be part of our brain keeping us mentally prepared – for example, concentrating on something for a long time and focusing our attention. Stress can be something that happens in a flash and is over very quickly ('acute' stress), or something that lasts longer and requires a more long-term physiological adaption (chronic stress).

If we think back over the last month or so, we'll probably be able to think of lots of different examples of things that we have found stressful. So, for example, stepping out into the road and then realizing we are about to be hit by a bus triggers what we might call an acute (short-term) stress reaction (that 'fight or flight' response again) which prepares us to jump out of the way. But living or working under a lot of pressure to get more done in the time we have than is realistically possible will trigger a more chronic (long-term) response as our body tries to focus our attention over long periods of time and work harder and faster. And the nature of stress means that even things we might not think of as 'stressful' do in fact produce a stress response in our body. A job that involves a lot of driving is actually very stressful, even on those days when the roads are clear and we are not running late, simply because of all the attention and concentration that driving requires.

Often, however, the most difficult causes of stress come from a third source. These are psychological and social triggers that are around us all the time in twenty-first-century life. They are more to do with situations that we *perceive* might happen and the emotional reaction we have as a result than with actual real-life disaster scenarios. So, everyday things can become a source of stress if we are pushing the limits. Being slightly late leaving for a meeting makes us worry and rush in case we miss it – that is a source of stress; trying to keep several things in our mind that we know we mustn't forget – that is stress; carrying responsibility for lots of different things such as our job, our children, our family – that is stress! Emotional stress responses occur when our brain pushes our body into responding to things that have not even happened yet. When our brain detects a set of things going on around us which *might* lead to a bad outcome, it triggers anxiety and a stress response almost as bad as if that most dreaded thing really had happened. In fact, sometimes it can feel even worse than if it actually had happened. How many of us have experienced how stressful it is to be driving somewhere to something we really shouldn't be late to, such as a vital work meeting, appointment of some kind, or to collect the children from school or nursery – and then been stuck in traffic? The stress response we experience then is often worse than the real result of being late. For some of us, these psychological triggers start to become overwhelming and the level of stress this can produce is huge as our body responds inappropriately to our worries and fears.

The physical response to stress

We'll look more at the emotional side later on, but for now let's concentrate on what happens physically when we are reacting to stress. Physiologically, the stress response is largely the same no matter what the trigger, because it uses the same system – something called the sympathetic nervous system. This is one of a set of nervous systems that operate automatically to try to keep things in our body in order. The sympathetic nervous system, roughly speaking, puts our body in a state in which we would be able to respond to any kind of danger or demand. So, it controls the fight or flight reflex but also responds to the more general or chronic stresses that we often find ourselves under. At the same time, it inhibits the action of another system working in our body called the parasympathetic system. This one keeps our body ticking over in the non-emergency moments and controls functions such as digestion. Activity in this system slows down when the sympathetic (stress) system is activated so that attention and resources are directed to where they are immediately required (or might be required).

So, when our brain identifies that something significant is happening, or might be about to happen, it triggers the sympathetic nervous system. This system is really a cascade of hormones and chemical messengers, each triggering the release of the next down the line. Each hormone or messenger released causes changes in the way our body is working. For example, when the sympathetic system is triggered, the combination of hormones causes glucose to be released into the blood as ready energy for our muscles, our heart rate to increase in order to deliver that glucose to where it is needed, and our breathing rate to go up so that we are flooded with oxygen and ready to react. Meanwhile, our parasympathetic system is slowed down, meaning that digestion and other functions are put on hold.

The stress response is a very complicated system made up of combinations of changes in lots of different places and with lots of different chemicals. It affects the body – but also the brain – not just in terms of how we think but at a real physiological level. The stress response seems to activate something called the serotoninergic system within the brain – that's the system that uses a chemical called serotonin to send messages, one which has been found to be very important in depression and anxiety amongst other things.[2] Stress also causes the release of other chemicals called peptides, which is all part of controlling our response and readying the body for action. Peptides are important in lots of areas of the body, including some parts of the brain, the immune system and even the reproductive system.

This means that the stress response really is one that affects our whole body. Although our emotions are often a significant component, just as much of the stress response comes from the real practical need that our body has to work harder and faster in order to meet the demands we are placing on it. In the same way that an engine has to work harder in order to move the car faster, the stress response revs our body faster in order to make sure that we keep up with the things we are trying to get done. This is not an optional response! If we are doing things hour after hour, day after day, that need us to concentrate or have us ready to react to anything that places us under physical or emotional pressure, we will experience a stress response to each of those things. Of course, everyone is different and just how aware we are of stress depends on many things to do with our personality, lifestyle and physical and mental health. We'll look at some of those things later. But, just like a car, if we constantly drive our body at high revs, we can expect to see some impact of that eventually.

3 When does stress start to become a problem?

Now that we know that stress is something real – and something that affects us physically as well as emotionally – it's important to know a bit about the specific kinds of impact that stress can have. Stress is blamed for all kinds of things, but what is the real evidence? What problems can stress cause, and what *kind* of stress is it that actually has these effects?

How the stress system is supposed to work

To understand better how stress can build up to a level that starts to cause problems, it's helpful first to look at how the stress system is supposed to work. Imagine for a minute that you were standing in a swimming pool, with most of the water drained out. We're going to use that image to represent the level of the various stress hormones in our body. Obviously it's a bit more complicated, but this image illustrates what happens when our stress levels start to rise. The water level is a bit like the level of all those stress hormones, and where it is now is the normal baseline level of your body's stress hormones – nice and low and very manageable (see figure 1).

Figure 1: Baseline level of stress

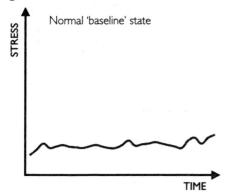

Now, most people agree that our body was designed to cope quite well with short-term (acute) stress. What happens then is that your brain triggers a response to the stress, which might look like a short spike on the graph (see figure 2). In our illustration this would be a bit like a wave in the swimming pool. Of course, with the water level at baseline, lapping calmly round your ankles, a wave isn't any problem and we cope with it just fine. Once the stress has resolved (remember it's only a momentary thing), hormone levels

Figure 2: Acute stress 'sparks'

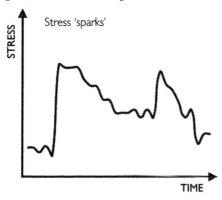

gradually come down again and very soon we are back at baseline. This pattern, with natural spikes that then die back down to normal, is quite healthy and unlikely to cause any problems. Normal everyday stresses which need us to respond happen quite naturally, and we even have the capacity to cope with something more major should it happen and keep on functioning just fine.

What happens when stress starts to build?

On the whole, trouble with stress starts when this natural rhythm of the system is interrupted. If you go back to the image of yourself standing in the swimming pool, you can imagine that the natural waves caused by stress spikes are fine if the water level is quite low, but there would be a 'crisis level' where, if the water were always that high, waves would start to be a real problem – the water could reach the kinds of levels where you might start to feel you were going under (see figure 3).

Figure 3: The 'crisis' level of stress

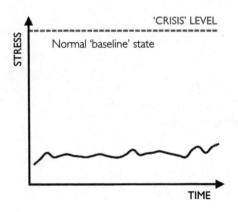

Two things can cause this to happen where stress is concerned. Remember that it takes some time for hormone levels to drop back down to baseline. If we are experiencing so much stress – that is, life is throwing so much at us that the next 'spike' happens before the last one resolves – the levels can easily start to get near to that crisis line (see figure 4). Most of us will have experienced days (or weeks!) like this, when one thing seems to come after another. Those are the days when one small thing at the end of the day can cause us to fly off the handle apparently irrationally. We come home and our partner asks us what's for dinner, and that question pushes us into an enormous rage as we feel totally overwhelmed by the unfair responsibility they expect us to shoulder. Or we drop a mug, and for some reason it just feels like too much and leaves us on the edge of tears. With the water levels raised, even the normal stresses of everyday life feel as if they push us close to the edge, and we are likely to find ourselves craving peace and quiet and some time to recharge our batteries.

Figure 4: Stress builds up to dangerously near crisis level

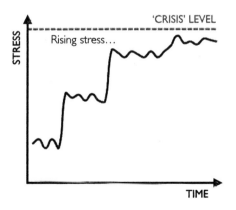

31

What we call 'recharging our batteries' is, of course, something that allows us to turn off the sympathetic system and chill out a bit, meaning that the water levels start to drop back down to our usual baseline. It is really important that this happens because it restores that natural 'ebb and flow' of the system. Unfortunately, however, this is often not what happens. If we do not have time to build in this rest and relaxation, if we are people who find relaxation challenging – or, of course, if the stresses bombarding us just keep on coming, then our system never gets this chance to 'reset'. As a result, something very important happens: in effect, our baseline level of stress hormones becomes chronically raised (see figure 5).

Figure 5: Baseline stress levels can become chronically raised

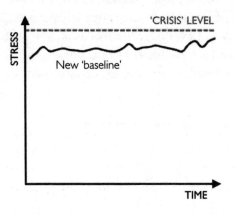

So, why does this matter, and what does this feel like in real life?

You probably won't notice your baseline stress gradually rising until it gets too close to that crisis level. Then you suddenly find that you are existing *all the time* with much higher water levels. You may well feel 'on the edge' because your baseline stress has become so high that even something relatively minor can easily push you not just into a difficult position but into a place where you risk a real crisis.

One person I have worked with is a typical example of this kind of pattern. He is a normal guy, working in an normal job, in a commuter town just outside Greater London. He came to speak to me after his doctor had told him that a physical problem he was suffering from was related to the stress he was under. 'The thing is,' he said to me, 'I just don't feel as if I am under that much stress. It's not as if I am a nuclear scientist, or a policeman, or anything like that. In fact, day by day I don't really find that the things I am facing are that stressful. But if I'm honest, I do feel on the edge. It's as if suddenly things that wouldn't have bothered me a few years ago have become big deals. So, if the kids are being difficult, I just can't handle it as well as I used to, and I am getting these thoughts flashing through my head about needing to escape or get away. I feel as if I'm constantly at the edge of my capacity to cope with whatever gets thrown at me, and it's a really uncomfortable feeling. I can't relax and now I am having trouble sleeping, which is making things even worse. I feel really weird because I don't see why I should have a problem, but, if I'm honest, it's starting to get scary because I don't know how to get out of feeling like this.'

This is an uncomfortable way to live life, and if this is you right now, you will be feeling pretty horribly aware of how stressed out you are. This kind of chronic rise in stress levels is very important because our body simply wasn't designed to exist under these kinds of conditions. As we'll see in the next chapter, if our body is exposed continually to raised levels of the stress hormones, it will have some physical and emotional impact on us, whether we are aware of it or not. Many of the physical effects in particular are things that build up over time, so it may be a long-term concern rather than something that we will notice right now. But, to be honest, most people know when they are living in this state, and it's not at all unusual.

In fact, twenty-first-century life can very easily push us into living with the kind of continual stress that can build up to this point. Many of us are living lives jam-packed with activities – be those work (as many of us work ever longer hours), family (just try getting a few children up, ready for school and out of the house on time five days a week!), relationship stresses, studying of some kind (many school children are now just as stressed out as their parents) or so-called leisure time ('work hard, play hard' might be fun, but it often isn't relaxing and can leave us totally exhausted as we try to pack too much in). Often it isn't that life is full of stress spikes, just that the general pace of life is so frantic that it becomes constant and consistently stressful, leaving little or no time for the vital relaxation which would restore the system back to baseline.

A woman I worked with explained to me the things that she felt were behind her own problems with stress. 'I know I am stressed-out a lot of the time,' she said, 'but I don't see what I can do about it. People always say I should do less or relax more – but when? If it's not getting the kids to school on time (which is always a nightmare), I am frantically cleaning, or cooking, or making costumes, or whatever the latest thing is they need. I've had to take on a part-time job to try to help bring some extra money in and that's really stressful because I'm constantly trying to work out how I can fit in the things I need to do for work around the edges of the things my kids need. I seem to spend most of my time feeling guilty. If I am working, I feel guilty and worry that my children need me, but if I am at home, I often am so aware of work that needs doing and I feel guilty for not doing that. I feel as if I am literally being pulled in several different directions and I am just not able to keep up with all the things I am supposed to be doing.'

Stressful events in life

For some of us, of course, the kind of stresses we are facing are not down to choices we have made. Life can throw things at us, and very often it seems to be totally unfair as lots of things all happen at once. Life events such as the death of someone close to us, moving house or even happy things that involve major changes to our life, such as getting married or leaving home, all trigger stress. In the late 1960s, a couple of psychiatrists worked through their notes on thousands of their patients and put together a list of stressful events that seemed to be linked to the chances of stress triggering illness in the people they were working with. The scale, which they then went on to test, gave each event a score. The idea was that you added up the total from each event you had experienced in the last year and this could give you an idea of the levels of stress you were under. Scores over about 150 seemed to indicate that you might be at risk of your stress causing you problems; at scores over 300 this was even more marked. You can see a list of some of the events and their scores in figure 6, overleaf.

Figure 6: Just some of the ratings given on the Holme and Rahe stress scale[1] (figures given are for adults)

Event	Score
Death of spouse	100
Divorce	73
Death of close member of the family	63
Personal injury/illness	53
Marriage	50
Loss of job	47
Retirement	45
Pregnancy	40
Major change in financial state	38
Death of a close friend	37
Change of job	37
Major change in responsibilities at work	29
Children leaving home	29
Starting or finishing school	26
Change in living conditions	25
Moving house	20
Change of school	20
Holiday	13
Christmas	12

Holme and Rahe's scale is interesting and it can give us an idea of roughly where we might expect our stress levels to be. But the truth is that different people experience stress very differently. The same event might be not much of a big deal to one person but an intolerable stress to someone else. The way we experience stress can be influenced by our personality, our aims and goals and the way we think. We also all notice stress at different levels. One person may feel dreadfully fraught and pressured, and another just think this is normal life, but both are at the same kind of stress level. Some people seem to thrive on stress and always like to be working towards something. The important thing to realize is that those people are just as likely to succumb to stress as anyone else.

How do you recognize when your stress levels are getting near that 'crisis' limit?

People differ in what first makes them realize there is a problem, but often it takes something reaching that crisis point before they start to do something about their stress. For some people it is a physical problem. Any doctor will tell you that many of the issues they see have their root in stress. Headaches, stomach pains, sexual problems, more serious issues such as irritable bowel syndrome (IBS) or heart problems – all these can be a wake-up call that we need to do something about our stress levels. Other people find that it is the emotional load that starts to push them over. Living constantly on the edge is exhausting and has an inevitable impact on our relationships, moods and emotions, and also on our ability to concentrate and perform effectively at work. Many people find that their stress suddenly brings them to a place where they become frightened that they simply will not be able to cope any longer and suddenly feel they are at very real risk of becoming a statistic of burn-out. If you recognize something of yourself in this chapter but haven't got to that point yet, fantastic! This is your chance to do something about your stress levels before they push you over the edge. If you have reached that point, then remember that you are not alone. Succumbing to stress is not a sign of weakness but a sign of being human. Your next challenge is to look at what it is in your life that has made you vulnerable to stress, so that you can protect yourself in the future.

4 The physical impact of stress

So far we've seen that stress is a physical reality as well as something that affects our emotions. It is much more than the kind of 'it's all in your mind' issue we often think it might be. Stress is something that, no matter how clever, resourceful or amazing we are, will affect us in some way because it is part of being alive. But what kind of problems can stress actually cause?

The problems caused by stress all stem from the fact that our stress system was actually designed to respond to *short-term* stress. Our bodies were simply not designed to operate with the levels of these hormones becoming raised over long periods of times. This is why chronic stress causes so many problems. It affects a vast array of different body systems and actions, with an impact that is often very complex and different for every individual. Chronic stress can affect a bewildering range of physical functions and has been linked to all kinds of illnesses, syndromes, signs and symptoms.

Physical issues related to stress

In some ways, the most serious physical results of stress are those that build up over time. The system that is most affected is the cardiovascular system – the heart and all the arteries and veins that carry blood to and from the muscles and organs that the heart supplies with blood. Stress stimulates the body to supply more blood to the major muscles, while organs – for example, those responsible for digestion – receive less blood. All this involves changes to the way the heart pumps, as well as changes to the blood vessels themselves. The bad news is that long-term stress stimulation of this system causes our blood pressure to rise (in an equally chronic, long-term way) as the vessels struggle to cope with the extra blood rushing through. It triggers changes in the way the heart muscle works, meaning that there is an increased risk of unusual or irregular beats. As if that weren't enough, chronic stress can also increase the risk of developing narrowing of the arteries (made all the worse, of course, if we tend to have a diet that is high in cholesterol and 'bad' fats). Chronic stress has, therefore, been linked to an increased risk of developing cardiovascular problems such as heart attacks and stroke. Acute stress can also trigger symptoms in these areas, bringing on conditions such as angina and chest pain. Meanwhile, of course, as the less important blood vessels receive less blood, stress can worsen illnesses related to poor circulation such as Reynaud's phenomenon, where people find that the blood supply to fingers and toes actually cuts off in cold weather, leaving their digits white, pale and painful.

Most of the problems stress causes in the cardiovascular system are related to the constant stimulation it receives. But remember that while the sympathetic system is overactive, it also effectively turns down the systems that control digestion. This means that stress very often causes some kind of digestive symptoms – from mild problems with indigestion to more serious conditions that require investigation and treatment. Chronic stress has been linked to conditions such as IBS, painful stomach cramps and problems with wind and constipation or diarrhoea. Stress can also contribute towards the development of stomach ulcers – both directly and because people often respond to stress by smoking or drinking too much alcohol, which can contribute to ulcers. An ulcer can be very painful and in some cases can become serious and cause secondary problems such as bleeding from the ulcer.

Stress can also cause muscular problems. When we are stressed, we are more likely to keep our muscles slightly tensed, meaning that they can become fatigued and painful. This effect may well contribute to another common symptom of stress – a type of headache called a tension-headache, where a mild or moderate pain around the head can feel like a band being tightened. This can be caused by muscles in the neck and at the back of the scalp being too tense and can be aggravated by poor posture. Chronic stress can also contribute to all kinds of other common muscle pains, including back and neck problems. So, although a bad back might be in part down to sitting badly, high stress levels will make it even worse.

As well as causing its own physical problems, stress can contribute towards the development of some illnesses. Studies have shown that long-term stress inhibits our immune system, meaning that we are more prone to coughs, colds and other bugs. In essence, we really can get 'run down'. Meanwhile some viruses – illnesses we have as children such as chickenpox – don't leave our body but remain dormant, waiting for a chance to re-emerge if our immune system is not working too well. Stress can trigger things such as shingles (which is what we get when the chickenpox virus re-emerges). Just how significant this impact on the immune system can be is still being investigated; it is even being linked to the development of some cancers.

The impact of stress on metabolism and eating

If you ask people what they do when they are stressed, one of the first things they are likely to mention is a change to their eating (or drinking!) habits. Stress has a significant impact on the way we break down and use our food. When the stress response is triggered, it causes various chemical processes to occur that result in glucose and certain types of fat molecules being released into the blood. This is to make sure we have the energy we might require to respond to the apparent threat. But if this happens over a long period of time, stress starts to cause more significant changes to the way we use and store foodstuffs such as fat and glucose. Blood levels of these molecules become chronically raised, and this can have serious consequences for our health.

We hear a lot about a type of diabetes that is becoming more and more common. Type 2 diabetes is caused by the cells in our body starting to become resistant to the insulin that is circulating. (People with Type 1 diabetes stop making insulin and therefore do not have enough circulating.) Insulin is absolutely vital, triggering our cells to take up the glucose they need in order to function. This process is also involved in getting fat cells to mop up and store any excess fat. In Type 2 diabetes, the cells stop responding to the insulin, meaning that glucose and fat levels in the blood rise – again contributing to cardiovascular disease. Type 2 diabetes is primarily caused by eating too much of the wrong things and gaining weight over a period of years. Chronic stress can add to this by causing our blood levels of glucose to be chronically higher anyway, which in itself gradually causes the cells to become less resistant to the insulin that is circulating. Type 2 diabetes is becoming a huge problem throughout the world. Previously referred to as 'adult onset' diabetes, it is now increasingly common in younger teenagers and even in children. Although this is often related to poor diet and rising levels of obesity, stress certainly has a part to play.

These metabolic changes don't just affect things inside our body; we may well notice changes in what we eat as well. Stress certainly affects our appetite, although exactly how it does so varies from person to person. Some people (apparently it's the minority – probably about one third of people overall) lose their appetites at the first sign of stress. Meanwhile, others overeat and tend to do so by snacking on high-sugar, high-energy foods that they are craving in order to gain the energy to respond to the demands placed on them. This can contribute to weight gain and often becomes part of a lifelong struggle with weight control.

Chronic stress also affects *where* we tend to put on weight. You will no doubt have heard about the difference between weight stored around the abdominal organs (round the middle, the classic 'apple' shape) as opposed to fat stored on the bottom and thighs (the 'pear' shape). For those people who eat more when they are stressed, the bad news is that this will stimulate fat to be laid down around the middle. This is the classic businessman's stomach – weight gain around the tummy! Unfortunately, fat stored around the middle is yet another risk factor contributing to cardiovascular problems.

Stress and pregnancy

The impact of stress in pregnancy is worth a special mention. When they fall pregnant, or are planning a pregnancy, most women make changes to their lifestyle in order to do everything they can for the health of the child. But how many people realize the impact stress can have? Evidence suggests that stress and anxiety are transmitted to the foetus as early as four months into the pregnancy, with levels of key stress hormones in the baby going up and down in tandem with levels in the mother's blood. Sometimes this stress can be linked to more serious problems, including birth defects, premature birth and pre-eclampsia.[1] In fact, amazingly, even stress in the six months *before conception* has been linked to a risk of premature birth. (A study of mothers in Denmark in 2008 looked at people who had experienced very serious stress caused by life events such as losing a partner or older child while pregnant.)

Of course, for most people this will not have any measurable impact, so don't panic – although high stress and anxiety levels in pregnancy have also been linked with having more irritable and difficult babies (something most parents are keen to avoid!). However, for those who have a personal or family history of some of these issues, it is sensible to look at how they can work on stress during this crucial time. And perhaps for all women considering pregnancy, it is worth taking stress as seriously as they do other factors such as their diet.

The physical reality of stress

This is an alarming wake-up call to the physical impact that chronic stress really can – and does – have on us. Far from being something minor that is linked to being slightly hysterical and not coping very well, stress is a physical reality with very real and serious short- and long-term outcomes. In fact, stress has been linked to and implicated in so many illnesses, diseases or negative outcomes that there simply isn't space to list them all. This chapter is really just a very brief overview.[2]

The take-home message from all of this is clear: we have to stop thinking that the 'best' people are those who can carry on in spite of lots of stress. Stress is a very real problem, a problem that affects everyone. It is something that we all need to be aware of, no matter how well we feel we may or may not cope when under stress. In fact, the more we tend to push ourselves and live life under stress, the more important it is for us to look at how we can manage that stress more effectively. It's for the sake of our health.

The good news is that we can do something about the impact stress is having on us. Look at the following true story of one person and the difference it made to his health when he changed the way he dealt with stress.

James is 36, with two young children and a busy job.

'I have to say that I thought getting help with stress was something that only weak people did – especially for men. It was not something I ever thought I would need to do. In my job, stress is something you just accept, and how you cope with that is taken as a sign of how good you are at your job. So, people who struggle are felt to be not up to it and often end up leaving the company. I never paid any attention to the stress I was under and I certainly never did anything to try to control the effect it had on my health.

'In the end, it was health issues that forced me to change that. I had been gaining weight for a while but thought nothing of it

– who doesn't gain weight! But I really didn't feel that great and I'd even had a couple of times when I had really bad chest pains – probably indigestion, but though I never admitted it to anyone, I was really worried. The final straw, though, was the headaches. I started to get really bad headaches – so bad that I just had to lie in a dark room until they had passed. It was a nightmare because I couldn't work when I had one so I was missing loads and had work stacking up behind me. I was trying to stay up late to catch up on work but that meant I missed out on sleep and made the headaches worse. In the end, I was finding that a headache would come on within less than an hour of starting work. I took a couple of weeks off but the minute I went back, the headaches came back. I went to the doctor, obviously, and they did some tests, but in the meantime they referred me to the practice nurse to talk about stress and stress management.

'It only actually took one session with the nurse to change everything. She explained all about stress, what it was and the effect it could have. I never realized how important it was to put in times to wind down and de-stress. I realized that everything I did was stressful – even in my spare time, the things I did were not relaxing. Neither I nor my wife ever took time out for ourselves – we were so busy focusing on other people.

'As a result of that session, I made some big decisions. I am a lot more careful now about the hours I work, and I spoke to my boss about the amount of work I was being expected to do at home in the evenings. I have started a hobby which really gets me out of the house and actually helps me to relax. I love having something in my life which I'm really passionate about but which isn't work! And it's made a difference to my life at home too as I am more relaxed with the family, so when I am there, it's more quality time. As for the headaches – well, I have to admit I was surprised. They stopped almost straight away and now I hardly ever have them. I

*feel loads better in myself and I guess I am just sorry that I didn't
realize sooner just how powerful stress could be.'*

5 The emotional impact of stress

So far we have looked at the various physical problems that stress can cause. But many of these are things we might not notice or things that build up over time. The most common visible sign or symptom of stress is often something to do with emotional or psychological factors. Here the impact varies along a spectrum, with minor changes in irritability at one end, right up to major breakdown and burn-out at the other.

In fact, to understand how stress affects us emotionally, we need to return to the happy and unhappy categories that I talked about in Chapter 2. To reiterate, many people like to think that where emotional problems (and certainly what we might call 'mental health' problems) are concerned, there are two sorts of people in the world. Most of us are lucky enough to be in the 'happy' group, people who do not have those kinds of issues and who consider themselves to be normal. Mental health crises are things that affect other people – the unlucky few who are in the other box, the 'problem' or 'not normal' box. We tend to think that these people, as a result of some quirk of genetics, personality or difficult start in life, will always have this tendency – this 'weakness' – to struggle with whatever the problem is, be it depression, anxiety or something more serious such as bipolar disorder or psychosis. Perhaps some people are unlucky enough to experience something extreme that can then catapult them from the healthy box into the unhealthy one for a time, but on the whole we can continue through life safe in the knowledge that mental health problems are things that affect other people.

Stress and mental health

In fact, the uncomfortable reality is that, although there are conditions such as schizophrenia which seem to affect certain people and have their own biological characteristics, in general, mental health is much more like a line, with 'healthy' at one end and 'unhealthy' at the other. Whoever we are and wherever we come from, life can sometimes throw things at us that we do not know how to cope with. This can push you down the line towards the level at which we might start to say that you have some kind of mental health problem. Some people have had experiences or a difficult start in life that might predispose them to struggle, but many mental health problems such as anxiety and depression are incredibly common, even in those people who have never had symptoms before. Statistics would tell us that in any given year one in four of us will develop a problem of this kind. Even looking at suicidal feelings – which you might consider to be a marker of a particularly extreme form of psychological distress – reveals that this kind of intense emotional pain is more common than we might think, with one in ten adults admitting that they have seriously considered suicide at some stage in their life.

Stress has been linked to almost every kind of mental health problem there is. In fact, it often precedes the development of depression and anxiety. (More about anxiety later, as it is one of the most common emotions to start to cause problems if you are operating under high stress.) Stress is a common cause of problems such as panic attacks or the kinds of psychological problem that can have a serious impact on everyday life – severe phobias or obsessive compulsive disorder, for example. If you are living on the edge of your capacity to cope, everyday stress can trigger emotions that feel very extreme and may feel out of control. Stress leads us to feel overwhelmed by the sheer volume of things that we are trying to keep on top of, and as a result we end up having to cope with a lot of negative emotions such as anxiety, as we desperately try to keep all those plates in the air. We have to accept that even for the strongest or most psychologically healthy of us, stress is one thing that can push us down the line towards problems if we are not very careful.

Part of our vulnerability to stress comes from what happens if we are simply bombarded with too many emotions. Emotions are complex things and very much a part of what it is to be human. They are a necessary and vital part of the way our brain is designed and we need them to help us to get through life successfully (see Chapter 7 for more). Very often, however, in our modern western lives, emotions – or, to be more specific, negative emotions – can start to cause very real problems. Being constantly inundated with negative emotions can cause us to turn to unhelpful things in order to try to help us to cope with them – an addiction or self-destructive behaviour, for example; something that actually makes us feel worse. Serious conditions such as eating disorders and self harm can develop as we desperately try to find a way to carry on with life in spite of difficult emotions. Stress, of course, is one of the major triggers for these kind of overwhelming emotions. It can cause an increase in emotions and also affect how vulnerable we are to them, making things feel more overwhelming and out of control.

Suppressing negative emotions

One of the reasons that we tend to struggle with the negative emotion thrown at us is the way that we often instinctively respond. Particularly if they are under stress, many people have a tendency to suppress negative emotions rather than deal with them in the moment they occur. Of course, suppressing emotions is something that all adults have to do to some degree. Some people would even argue it is a necessary skill to gain with maturity. In adult life, it can be inappropriate to react immediately and vocally to every emotion we experience. We have to be able to control our emotions in certain circumstances. In the short term, this can even be a positive coping strategy to deal with a difficult situation – in effect, to put that feeling to one side and deal with it later when there is more time and when it is more appropriate. Some jobs in particular require this kind of emotional maturity – jobs that involve working with children such as teaching or childcare, jobs where you support people who are themselves struggling with difficult emotions, or jobs where certain behaviour and standards are very important. However, the very same tendency to suppress emotions that can be a good thing in those contexts can quickly start to be a problem if we are experiencing a lot of stress.

The problem with chronically stressful situations is, in a nutshell, that there is never any time to give ourselves a chance to deal with an emotion or to work through what happened and how it made us feel. Most people in our current culture admit that they struggle to find times where they can wind down and take time to think through and assess things that have happened during the day or week. Indeed, one third of adults say that they never experience any time that is truly private and gives them the chance to think these kinds of things through. Meanwhile, although friendships are increasingly important as families now live further apart, many people find that their friendships are starting to lack the kind of depth that they really need in order to get support from them. So, although they might have loads of friends they would get together with for a laugh or a night on the town, many people struggle to think of who they would turn to if they were really in need. This lack of social support leads us to feel even more under pressure to find the solution within ourselves.

The problem with suppressing emotion is that it just doesn't work. In fact, a tendency to do this – and the extreme where people start to become unaware of the emotions that they are experiencing – has been linked to a whole host of emotional and psychological problems. Suppressed emotions tend not to stay suppressed. So, at moments when we feel vulnerable (often when we are on our own, tired or trying to rest and relax), those emotions re-emerge. This means that people often find themselves struggling with what can be called 'free floating' emotions – emotions with no apparent trigger in that moment. This constant low-level negative emotion then affects our thinking and can lead us to start to make irrational leaps in our thinking that emphasize the negative and ignore positives. All of these things can trigger a new problem or worsen an existing tendency towards a mental health issue.

The vicious cycle of stress

So, one way in which stress has its emotional impact is related to the way it makes us more likely to act or think in certain ways. There are also physiological reasons why our brains, under stress, are more likely to react in certain ways. Stress hormones can affect the parts of the brain that moderate and regulate mood, and there is good evidence that chronic stress can genuinely affect the way our brain responds to the world around us, making us more prone to low moods and problems with motivation. Stress also contributes to other problems such as insomnia (see Chapter 17) which can worsen psychological disorders, and it is very easy to end up in a vicious cycle. Imagine, for example, the following situation:

Alex is 38 and works in what you might call a pretty normal managerial job. However, recently she has been under a lot of pressure and given new responsibilities which she struggles to get done alongside her usual work. Because of this she has found herself starting to struggle with anxiety and she finds it really hard to switch off from her work and not to worry about it when she should be doing other things. She used to use other things to help her switch off – things such as going to the gym, cinema or meeting up with friends. But now her job means that she has to spend extra time working in the evenings, and if she does arrange to go out, she feels guilty for not working so she just doesn't go. She often intends to work in the evenings but is too exhausted so ends up slumped in front of the TV watching whatever's on and eating. She's also noticed that she is drinking more than usual on her own at home – what used to be the occasional glass doesn't seem to help her relax any more, and she notices with alarm how easy it is to be getting through several bottles of wine a week. Recently she's started feeling kind of odd – very tearful and emotional. She finds herself having thoughts that she cannot cope and sometimes she just wants to run away and hide – but she knows she can't. On top of everything else, she is now having trouble sleeping, which is just making everything worse. She really wonders how long she will be able to keep going like this.

Does that sound familiar? It is all too easy for a stressful situation – be it at work or elsewhere – to trigger difficult emotions and very quickly push us into a position where we find we are struggling to cope. Often our own reactions to that then make things worse. So, a stressful job causes stress and triggers emotion, but the same stressful job means that there is never time for us to deal with or express that emotion. The same stressful job means that when we are not working, either we are frantically keeping up with the other chores that life presents – shopping, cleaning, basic things – or we are out trying to have fun. And that is not exactly a time when we want to be having heart-to-hearts and going over all the things that made us feel so dreadful that week – we want to escape it all and forget. So, we go out, we have fun, maybe we end up drinking a bit too much or trying something else in order to get away from the realities of our day-to-day life. All too soon it is time to be back at work, often worn out as a result of lack of sleep over our hectic weekend, and those emotions simply become part of the pool of things we have not had a chance to deal with. But at the times when we are vulnerable – perhaps those moments after a long busy day when we are finally on our own, perhaps the long hours at night when we are lying awake, unable to switch off and get to sleep – then those emotions can come flooding back and leave us feeling totally overwhelmed and out of control.

Of course, this also means that people experiencing chronic stress can be at a heightened risk of slipping into unfortunate strategies to try to cope with all of that emotion day to day. The occasional glass of wine to relax can quickly become something more serious, or people can start to develop a problem with self harm, which so often begins in someone desperately trying to cope with what they are feeling and go on as normal. Meanwhile, disruption to appetite, combined with this need to find a way to cope with what life is throwing at them, can contribute towards the development of eating disorders. On top of all that, chronic stress can seriously affect sleep. As well as causing its own problems as we get more and more tired, insomnia tends to magnify any existing problems and again increases the risk that we might turn to something else in order to try to cope.

In essence, chronic stress pushes our capacity to cope to the absolute limit, and as a result reveals any inherent weak points in our personality, relationships, thinking style, beliefs or the way we deal with difficult emotions. If we're honest, most of us would admit that although we are normally fairly stable, a bad day can push us so that we behave like someone we barely recognize! Stress does this, pushing our resources and forcing us to the very edge of what it is to be us. Even though this often resolves in time as the source of stress goes away, the risk is that for some of us – who for whatever reason are particularly vulnerable (more in later chapters) – all of this goes on to trigger a serious emotional or psychological problem.

Remember, these things are much more common than you might imagine! Don't make the mistake of thinking you are immune to emotional problems. Just as we take measures to think about our physical health and try to make changes to keep ourselves healthy, it is vital that we do not neglect our emotional well-being. And just like issues relating to our physical health, this is particularly important if we are under a lot of stress. Stress is like a magnifying glass: it takes any potential weakness in our psychological make-up and makes it seem much bigger!

Here's the experience of one woman who knew all too well the impact stress was having on her emotions. Mary is 32. She's single and works as a PA.

'I think for me stress has always been something that has affected me. Even when I was in school I struggled with it – I remember having to take time off during exams, and having panic attacks a lot. The teachers always said I was "highly strung" and I guess I have carried that label with me all my life. In work situations, I have always avoided stressful stuff because I know I don't handle it very well and I am worried about flaking out. I have missed out on promotions and so on, and although I have been in this job for ages and watched other people move up the ladder, I have never been offered anything. But that's not their fault because I think I took the job because I knew it wouldn't be too much for me.

'The trouble is I have a pattern of stress making me stop what I am doing. When I was at school they put me in for my exams and I was expected to do well, but what actually happened was that I fell ill and ended up missing most and doing really badly in the exams I did sit. They said that the illness was stress – I don't really remember much about it now but I guess it probably was that. In the end, I left school and got a job as a secretary – I taught myself a lot of the skills and did an Open University course at home. That all went fine until they did promote me – to a manager's post that meant I was running a small office and in charge of a few staff. I did OK at first, but in the end I couldn't handle the stress and

I went off on long-term sick leave. I just felt really tearful all the time and the anxiety was dreadful – even something little such as going to the shops left me feeling sick with fear.

'I decided to try and get some help after hearing a piece about stress on the television. I had always thought that this was just part of me – that I was weak in some way or a failure. But it made me realize that there might be something I could do about it – to change the effect stress had on me. I was fed up of it holding me back and I wanted to give it everything I had to see if I could change. I was referred to see a CBT [Cognitive Behavioural Therapy] practitioner, and started a process of looking at the way I was thinking and the things I believed about myself. I have to say it was hard work and the results weren't immediate, but now, a year or so on, I definitely see a difference in myself. It really made me challenge some of the assumptions I made and understand how things were affecting me. It's made me feel much more in control – and although I am still someone who is quite emotional, I feel much more able to handle it. I am thinking a lot about my future and planning to do some extra training so that I can get a better job. I think in the long run it will totally change my life.'

6 Why are you reading this book?

We end part one of this book, then, with a pretty good idea of what stress is and the way that it can affect us, in the short and long term. In the next part, we'll look a bit more at some of the common issues that are associated with stress and start to think about what we can do in order to protect ourselves from the health problems it can cause.

Before we move on though, now is a good time to think about why you are reading this book and what you want to get out of it. Whoever you are and however you got hold of this book, the chances are you are concerned about the issue of stress – either for yourself or for someone else. It may be that you are already experiencing some difficulties – physical or emotional – as a result of stress. Or you may have bought the book thinking of someone else who you feel sure is suffering as a result of stress. Some of you may have come to this point because you are aware of the stress you are under, perhaps as an inescapable part of the job you do or the lifestyle you lead. What all of us who meet here on this page have in common is that we are people who want to avoid the negative impact stress can have on our lives and the lives of those around us.

Stress and doing less

There is another issue that is important to mention because

it concerns a lot of the people I talk to about stress. In fact, I've already mentioned it in passing. Most people are very reluctant to come to see me, feeling that they know what I will say about stress and that it is something they don't want to hear. If stress is an issue for you, then to the people around you there seems one obvious solution: cut back on what you are doing and just do less! But the people who come to me struggle with that response. Some, quite rightly, point out that they are not doing *that* much – it's just that it seems to affect them particularly strongly. Others are simply not in a position where they can jettison the cause of their stress. If you are caring for an elderly relative, a young child or someone who is chronically ill, you cannot simply stop doing it because it makes your life stressful. And, particularly in difficult times, many people are forced to live lives in which they do pack things in, just to stay financially afloat. It isn't their choice but they are stuck with it. Finally, and, if we're honest, this fits for a lot of us, many people I talk to just don't want to do less! They're doing the things they do because they enjoy them and are passionate about them. So, the stressful job, the out-of-hours volunteering, juggling work and family life – lots of us do those things because we like to live that way. As one person explained to me, 'I did try doing a less stressful job. I did it and I was good at it, and it worked, kind of. People said to me that I seemed much less stressed, much more healthy. But I was bored. And I didn't feel fulfilled. So I only lasted a year.'

Learning to handle stress well

The reality is that, for whatever reason, a lot of us find ourselves needing to learn to cope with situations in which stress is thrown at us, often on a daily basis. If you are one of those people, then this book is for you. It is true that your problems with stress would probably improve if you did less. However, if you want, intend or need to continue living on the edge, then it is vital that you learn how to handle stress well. On top of that, you may well find it helpful to look at some things that might make you more prone to stress. There may be things about the way you think, or about the way you handle certain emotions or situations, that you might be able to change in order to make you more effective at resisting the impact of stress. This is particularly key if you are one of those people who thinks that they don't actually do *that* much, but seem always to end up fighting stress. It may be that there is something about the way you approach life that makes you more prone to stress. Finally, and most importantly, if there is one thing that anyone who wants to live a life impacted by stress must learn – one golden rule – it's this: you must find an effective way to take time out and relax!

There is a very good reason why all this is so important. Very often the kinds of people who are most at risk of stress are those who genuinely have a great deal of potential. They are often academically clever, as well as resourceful and capable. They are driven, but also organized and capable of achieving success. Perhaps most importantly, they are passionate people who tend genuinely to care about what they do and want to do it well. This makes them very valuable people to have around. We might say that those people were created with that gift of being able to get things done and achieve a lot. Certainly these people are not likely to be limited in life by their ability. Throughout their life and work, they will improve their skills and become more efficient and able in what they do, but if something is going to stop them from progressing, or cause them problems, it is unlikely to be related to how good they are at what they do. The reality is that the thing most likely to hold you back if you are in this group is the way you handle the stress and pressure that you will most likely find yourself under.

How many times have you heard a story like this one?

John is in his thirties and works for a large well-known company. He has always done pretty well at whatever he has put his mind to, coming out of school with good grades and getting a good degree. After university he wanted to find a job that challenged him, so he started a management training scheme and, true to form, did pretty well, eventually being offered the job he still does now. He enjoys work and likes the buzz of deadlines, but he struggles with the long hours and the demands his work places on him. He wanted to do something worthwhile, so he has also become involved with volunteering at a local scout group. That is hard work too, but they really need him: there aren't many people to run it and he is very aware that if he didn't turn up one week, it probably wouldn't happen. John wants to enjoy what he is doing, and people around him tell him that he is doing really well, but lately he has started to find it all a bit of a strain. He worries a lot about decisions he has made at work, and often works late into the night trying to get reports done really well so that his boss will be happy. He used to go out a lot to meet friends but recently there hasn't been time, so since he started work, his only friends are the people he sees there. He tries not to show it but, if he's honest, he is starting to struggle with the pressure. He worries about losing his job – his company has laid some people off recently – and he also finds the scout group preying on his mind because he is so aware of how much it depends on him. He has started to have trouble sleeping and finds he wakes early in the morning and cannot get back to sleep, although at least this means he gets into work early, which makes a good impression. Recently he's had to see the doctor about some stomach trouble he's been having, and he knows he is drinking too much, but he just needs to wind down sometimes after a hard day.

That story isn't a real one, but it is based on elements that are common to almost all the experiences I have heard from people who are struggling with stress. All are people who have great potential and are very able at what they do. This means they are greatly in demand, but often they do not share the level of belief in themselves that others seem to have, which means they are prone to anxiety. Often they take on lots of different responsibilities and find themselves juggling these many demands on their time. As a result, time for themselves and things they used to do for fun gets pushed out or just becomes yet another demand.

Some people who live life like this – and there are lots of us! – manage to carry on with this level of stress. But for most, the level of stress life places them under will take its toll. People differ in how much they are able to carry and in what it is that pushes them outside their coping zone. Some people find that something stops them in their tracks fairly early on and makes them reassess what they are doing. Often they are forced to give up some of the things they love in order to create some time to recover. Some people show a pattern of this: taking lots on and throwing themselves into things, then struggling with stress and having to cut back. You may know someone like this or recognize it in yourself. The tragedy is that sometimes these people are labelled as unreliable, weak or 'over-emotional' as a result. They may be given less responsibility or overlooked for promotion because of their apparent inability to 'take the pressure'. But the fact is that there is nothing wrong with their abilities; they just need to learn how to deal with stress so that their potential can be properly released. People like John live life on a tightrope, working hard each day to keep upright but knowing at the back of their mind that they are pushing themselves to the limit. It's a hard way to live.

So, how do you know if you are in that place right now?

What are the early warning signs and symptoms of stress? You can see a list of some of the common signs in figure 7 on the next page. But very often you can trust your own judgment. You probably know in your heart of hearts if you are pushing the limits. Watch for the fleeting thoughts that show that you are at the edge of what you can handle. You might find yourself worrying about the responsibility you are under, or thinking, even for a moment, that you cannot cope. Or you might see other emotional signs of the strain you are under. Some people find that they become more emotional, reacting to things that wouldn't usually get to them. Remember, if your stress baseline has been raised so it is right near the crisis zone, everyday little things might feel much more major. People might say that you are over reacting, or you might feel that yourself. The chances are that you are just a human being struggling with too much stress.

For some people, of course, physical issues are the first thing to come to a head. Starting to find that you are frequently unwell – whatever form that takes – can quickly become a vicious cycle as you become under further pressure because you are missing things. Do act fast if you suspect, or are told, that stress might be a contributing factor. Remember, it is not

Figure 7: Early warning signs of stress

Physical signs/symptoms	Emotional signs/symptoms
Frequent headaches	Feeling more tearful or angry than usual
Problems with indigestion or irritable bowel syndrome	Panic attacks
Worsening of conditions such as eczema	Emotions feeling out of control
Sweating or shaking at times when you are under pressure	Mood swings
Chest pains/rapid heartbeat	Withdrawing from friends/ family – feeling you want to be on your own more than usual
Hyperventilation (over-breathing)	Feeling agitated and unable to relax
Sleep problems (struggling to get to sleep or waking in the night)	Struggling to switch off your thoughts/worries
Frequent minor illnesses such as colds	Inability to concentrate/ plan things in the way you normally can
Loss of sex drive/decreased interest in sex	Feeling more sensitive than usual to criticism or problems at work and at home

a sign of weakness to find that stress is having an impact on you. Often people ignore those physical warning signs – men especially – or see them as annoying niggles that get in the way instead of genuine and important warnings that your body is under strain. Dealing more effectively with stress needn't be about giving things up; it is about changing the way you do things, but doing so to become *more* productive, not less! Ultimately, learning how to handle stress will make you more effective, more able, and help you to carry more, not less.

PART 2

All about you

WHAT MAKES SOME PEOPLE PARTICULARLY VULNERABLE TO STRESS?

7 I feel, therefore I am! Emotions and how they relate to stress

In part 1 we looked at some background information about stress: what it is and what it can do to us. Stress can come from a number of different sources, and what might be stressful to one person might not be to another. This section is all about the things that make us different from one another and, importantly, how those things can make some of us more prone to problems with stress. We'll start by looking in more detail at an issue we explored in Chapter 5: the way we respond to and deal with negative emotions.

How emotions are supposed to work

In order to understand exactly how our emotions can start to cause us problems, it is important to have an idea of the way emotions are meant to work. People often think that emotions interrupt good rational thought and make us behave in less sensible ways. So, we say things such as 'Don't be so emotional', and scoff at those who 'go by their emotions'. Characters depicted in films and TV who do not have emotions (think Spock in *Star Trek*: 'Emotions are alien to me, I'm a scientist'; or the Terminator: 'I know now why you cry, but it is something I can never do') are often supposed to be more logical, more wise, more able as a result. Emotions are seen as something faintly quaint, a let-down to the human species. The reality is far from this. In fact, emotions are critical to the way our brain works.

Think about the last time you felt a certain emotion – say, anxiety. Chances are there are four things that you were experiencing, which all together make you identify it as a time when you had that emotion. First of all there was some kind of **physical feeling**. Some emotions have stronger and more obvious physical characteristics than others. Anxiety, for example, tends to involve feeling fidgety, butterflies in the stomach or maybe feeling sick, whereas other emotions such as sadness are harder to define in terms of the physical feelings they trigger. The next thing is that an emotion affects your **thoughts**. Each emotion tends to have characteristic thoughts that go with it. These might be different for different people. Anxiety tends to trigger thoughts linked with uncertainty – worries about what might happen. The third feature of an emotion is that it tends to **make us *do* something** – or at least *want* to do something. So, continuing to use anxiety as an example: if you are feeling anxious, you probably find it hard to sit still. Anxiety makes us want to move around, and it might trigger feelings of wanting to escape or run away. Finally, an emotional experience has a fourth characteristic – something really quite hard to put your finger on or explain – **that elusive thing** that just makes us *know* we are experiencing an emotion.

It's interesting to note that different emotions have these different components in different measures. An emotion such as anger or frustration is very much about what it makes us want to do. We might find ourselves feeling totally out of control as we give in to the urge to yell, hit someone or just stamp our feet! Meanwhile, an emotion such as anxiety is very physical – and not in a very pleasant way. We might feel overwhelmed with the feeling of butterflies in our stomach to the degree that we feel sick. Some emotions are very strongly controlled and maintained by the thoughts that go with them, so it is impossible to imagine being worried without linking that to something you were worried about, to the thoughts you were having. In general, negative emotions tend to be quite clearly defined in terms of one or more of these four features. It is interesting that positive emotions such as happiness or joy are so much less specific. These emotions have that strange fourth factor as the dominant thing we notice. We can clearly say when we have felt happy or joyful, but it is hard to define exactly what it was about the way we were feeling that makes us say it was happiness or joy.

All of these different features of emotion give us some vital clues to what their overall role is. The study of emotions is a field where psychology, neuroscience, sociology and many other disciplines all come together, and one area all have questioned is what emotions do – in particular negative emotions, which are those that tend to cause all the problems. On the whole, there are three functions for those emotions that most experts agree on.

The first thing is that emotions are about **drawing our attention to something**. Our brain is constantly scanning the world around it, looking for things going on that might be significant to a goal we have – a general one such as staying alive, or something more specific such as getting a report in on time. If our brain identifies something significant happening – say, we have stepped out into the road and a bus is coming right at us – then it triggers an emotion as part of drawing our attention to the fact that something is happening that might need us to take action. This is particularly true about emotions that have a strong physical component such as anxiety and anger. In fact, one expert, writing in the nineteenth century, went as far as to say that what we call an emotion *is* our experience of those physical changes.[1]

The second function that emotions have is to make sure that we **do something**. Emotions are a bit like special kinds of reflexes. If you reach into the oven to get something out and part of your hand not covered by the oven glove accidentally touches the metal side, you will automatically and without thinking jerk your hand away. This is a physical reflex response. Emotions act in a similar way. Listen to the way one expert put it: 'The human body has at its disposal two methods by which it can change its circumstances. It can do so by altering behaviour, causing for example shivering or reflexes. Alternatively it can resolve the predicament by inducing physiological states that lead individuals to act in a certain way.'[2] So, an emotion changes something about our physical state that makes us much more likely to act in a certain way – a way that is likely to resolve whatever the significant situation is. When we have walked out in front of the bus, the emotion anxiety (or more likely panic!) makes us instinctively want to jump back out of the way. In fact, there is evidence that in the case of strong emotions triggered by very significant or risky situations, the brain can actually bypass the part where thinking occurs and just trigger a physical response. So, without thinking about it, we jump back to safety, responding without having to waste valuable time thinking about whether we should. This physical push to act in a certain way can be very strong – just think about how hard it is not to run away if you are scared of something –

72

and is often what makes certain emotions so hard to ignore.

Finally, emotions have a very influential role in our **decision-making**. Very few of our day-to-day decisions can be made by mathematical analysis of the facts. Even if they could, who has time to approach decisions in that way? Attempts to create computer models that think like humans find that without something that does a similar job to emotions to simplify decision-making, the computer becomes overwhelmed by simple decisions. In a similar way, humans who have had brain injuries that appear to have impaired their emotions struggle terribly with the simple decisions of everyday life. Emotions seem to colour our perception of an option, so if one option is associated with a negative emotion such as anxiety, we are much less likely to consider it. This is worth being aware of because it can make decisions very hard if one option is associated with a very strong emotion, even though it is probably what we want to do. So taking an exam might trigger a lot of anxiety but be something we need to do in order to pass a course. That kind of decision can become very stressful because it almost requires over riding the warning that the emotion is giving.

Suppressing emotions

So, emotions are automatic things. They are not optional and they are not something we could live without. This is important because too often we treat emotions as if they *should* be optional! We wish we didn't feel an emotion, or we feel it is inconvenient to feel it, so we try to suppress it; we try to deny that it is there. Our response is to criticize ourselves and wish that we didn't feel that way, perhaps adding guilt to the emotional mix as we struggle with the fact that we reacted in that way. But although we can control how we react and what we do as a result, *having* an emotion is not something we can control. Let's look at example. Say a friend has just announced that they are getting married. What we want to feel is joy and happiness for them but, for some reason that we are not quite sure of, what we actually find ourselves feeling is a very negative emotion such as jealousy or sadness. Now we have a choice about how we deal with an emotion which, if we were honest, we would rather not be feeling. Very often what people do in this kind of situation is try desperately hard not to feel it. They very much wish that they didn't and push it right down in the hope that it will go away. But, of course, it doesn't; in fact, it seems to bubble to the surface more and more, and soon it will become an issue that they will have to deal with one way or another. Suppressing emotions rarely works. The way to work with an emotion like that, uncomfortable as it may be, is to look at why it has been triggered in the first place and deal with the perhaps uncomfortable realities that underlie it. So, if you want to get rid of your uncomfortable emotion, you have to look at where it comes from. Only then, when you have processed the things that are causing it to be triggered, will it start to go away.

In fact, this kind of instinctive suppression of emotions is very often at the root of a more serious problem. If we start habitually to suppress emotions that we do not know how to deal with, this pattern of suppressing them becomes less of a short-term solution and more of a habit. In effect, we start to treat emotions as if they are awkward things that we would rather not have. So, faced with a situation that leaves us feeling really upset or anxious, we take a deep breath, 'pull ourselves together' and carry on regardless. What happens to that emotion? If only it did what we wanted and just dwindled away to nothing! Remember, an emotion's job is to get our attention! If we were given the job of getting someone's attention and their first reaction was to ignore us, would we go away? No, we'd keep on catching them whenever we could and reminding them that we were there until they finally paid attention! Negative emotions do not generally go away until we have worked through whatever triggered them in the first place.

Trying to suppress negative emotions is a bit like putting an angry cat in a box. We might manage to get it in and shut the lid, and there might be no outward signs that it is there, but it *is* there, and from time to time we will know it is as we hear angry yowls or maybe see the occasional paw break out. All that time it is in there it gets more and more angry, and at some point, eventually, we will have to open the box. This kind of delayed emotional attack is often both painful and overwhelming.

This is exactly what happens when we are under long-term stress. We start automatically to suppress some emotions – often those that are painful, unpleasant, unwanted or inconvenient. We're even more likely to do this if life is throwing a lot of us, so there are simply too many emotions for us to deal with in the time we have available. As we start habitually to suppress our emotions, we end up with a box full of these difficult, negative feelings that we have never processed or dealt with. They can become a bit like a bubbling pool of festering emotion that we carry around with us. Carrying this has various effects on us. Sometimes those feelings, which do emerge from time to time, can start to trigger worries that we have always had about who and what we are. Of course, this then triggers more emotions and fears, and can very quickly result in a lot of pressure for us to carry each day as those doubts and worries build up. We may find that we start to change in ourselves, becoming more withdrawn, quiet or subdued as we have to try not to react to anything in case those other feelings come flooding out.

Meanwhile, of course, all that effort is tiring, so we will find ourselves feeling more and more emotionally exhausted and worn out. Sometimes the effort of just talking to someone else can be too much, so we might start to avoid other people and become isolated. Being on our own then leaves us vulnerable to more emotions emerging. Bit by bit things can start to get really hard. On the surface we may look fine but gradually we will become all too aware of what we are carrying round underneath. As someone said to me once, 'I've just got to a stage where I don't know what to say if someone asks me how I am. The answer isn't "fine" because I am not. But I am still managing just about OK. The thing is there is so much under the surface that not even I know how I am any more – I just get on with being. So I have to avoid other people in case they ask me how I am because I guess the honest answer is that I am not sure that I want to know.'

Emotional sparks and emotional fires

So, something as simple as suppressing emotions can easily cause them to become a problem in their own right. The other common cause of problems with emotions is the way that they can grow. Remember, emotions as they are supposed to work are short-term triggers – like warning flags that signal there is something you need to pay attention to.

I like to think of them as emotion sparks – you can see them at the top of figure 8. Sparks of emotion are not optional. They are designed to grab our attention so that we address the potentially significant thing that is going on around us. They act a bit like smoke alarms, warning us that there might be something serious going on. Once we have realized that, they die out – they have done their job.

The trouble is that many of us are dealing with something quite different – emotional fires. Emotional fires start when we move into the bottom half of the diagram – when that initial spark of emotion seems to ignite something else and start a much bigger reaction.

Figure 8: Emotion sparks and emotional fires

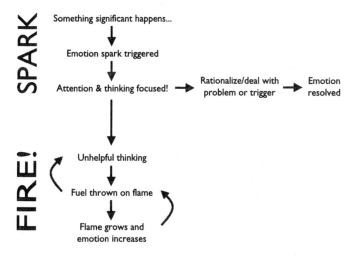

How do emotional fires start? In essence, they happen when something about the kind of person we are and the way we approach the world makes us more prone to certain unhelpful ways of thinking (these are covered in detail in Chapter 10). Remember, a key part of an emotional experience is the thoughts that it triggers – thoughts that start us off analysing what caused the emotion in the first place. Too often, however, the initial thoughts linked with the emotion spark can then trigger a load of other, less helpful thoughts. Imagine your brain triggers an emotion to alert you to the fact that you have not yet finished a report due in tomorrow. You feel anxious and find yourself thinking about the report, how it needs doing, what might happen if you cannot get it finished in time. But often these anxious thoughts can then trigger others. What about that other project you have to work on? What if you end up late with that one too? What if your boss just thinks you are totally useless? Remember how you did that report last week and he thought it was dreadful? What if that happens again?

Sometimes these thoughts can trigger weaknesses in what you think of yourself (see Chapter 11 on self-esteem) – 'I'm so useless, I can never get anything done on time!' or 'I always make a hash of these things!' – or beliefs and pressures that we put on ourselves – 'I must get everything right or I am not good enough!' or 'I should be able to get this done without any help.' The key thing is that these kinds of thoughts are a bit like kindling. If you are prone to thinking in certain ways, then it is rather like lighting a match in the middle of a dry forest in a hot summer. One tiny spark of emotion can easily set fire to these thoughts, creating a much bigger emotion that is more difficult to deal with.

Looking at the spark/fire model of emotions, we can quickly see that there are two ways in which emotions could start to become problematic and leave us vulnerable to trying to suppress them. The first is if there are just too many – if our brain is triggering too many sparks. This can happen if something about the way we live our life means we have a lot of rules or goals that our brain is trying to keep track of. They may be things we believe about ourselves or things that are related to the world around us, but they mean our brain is constantly having to grab our attention, resulting in a lot of emotion sparks. The second problem is if emotion sparks are then building up into emotional fires. This happens if, again as a result of what life has taught us so far, we tend to think in certain ways or hold certain beliefs about the world that act in a negative way, building up blazes of negative emotion. We'll look at this in more detail in Chapter 10.

Understanding our emotions enables us to start the journey of changing the way stress affects us. Ultimately though, the key to managing our emotions is to learn to treat them as what they are: useful warning flags that alert our attention to things and help to colour our judgments. But we are always going to struggle with this if our emotions are out of control. It's much better to prevent fires than to have to fight them. The next step, therefore, is to move on and look at the patterns of thinking and belief that can be behind troublesome emotions.

8 Anxiety: fighting the fires

Before we move on from looking at how negative emotions affect us, we need to look at one example of an emotion that we could say causes more problems than any other. This emotion is at the root of many mental health problems, including obsessive compulsive disorder and phobias, and it is even implicated in other conditions such as eating disorders and self-harm. It can cause and trigger other problems but it can also be the problem itself. It has the power to control our lives and to back us into a corner as we retreat ever further away from things that seem to make it worse. It is the only emotion to have its own category in the clinical manual used by psychologists to diagnose psychological illnesses. Most importantly, because of the hormones and chemical reactions it triggers, it is one of the emotions most strongly linked with stress. It is anxiety.

Anxiety is a very powerful and unpleasant emotion. Of course, there are good reasons for this. If emotions in general are designed to trigger our attention, perhaps more than any other anxiety needs to be something that *forces* us to pay attention. Anxiety is triggered when there is a chance that a situation playing out around us will lead to an outcome that is unwanted for us or that risks something very precious to us. Anxiety can be a very intense, instant reaction that causes us to react instinctively without thinking – for example, if we (or someone we care about) are in personal danger. Or it can be something that burns more slowly in the background: a base level of unpleasant emotion that never quite goes away.

Anxiety can have a clear root cause and trigger. Someone who has been in a bad car accident might struggle with severe anxiety about driving a car again, suffer panic attacks when on motorways and find it takes a lot of work to get back into driving again. Just as often, however, anxiety can be apparently inexplicable, as in the case of bizarre but very powerful phobias.

Anxiety and the worst case scenario

The first step in understanding anxiety is to look at how it forms and at something quite unique in the way we instinctively respond to it that tends to make things much worse. At the root of any episode of anxiety is what I call the worst case scenario (WCS) – that thing that we fear might happen, that we dread happening, that we want to stop happening. So we become anxious because there is something we are worried might happen – an essential element for anxiety is uncertainty. Anxiety is triggered when our brain detects that something happening around us, or something we are doing, might be linked to increasing the risk of this WCS happening. Sometimes this is because we have had a bad experience of it happening before. Sometimes it is an automatic instinctive fear that something bad will happen. Or it has been suggested that a tendency to be scared of some things is innate – being scared of spiders or snakes, for example. We don't know why, and we don't have to have had a bad experience ourselves, we just know that something bad might happen if we go near them.

The classic response to fear is to start straight away to avoid the thing that has been linked in our minds with the WCS. I'll use an example from my own life to show what I mean. When I was about seven, I was stuck in a lift with my family during a power cut in a hotel in Italy. It was a pretty short experience – my parents say it actually lasted only minutes – but I still remember it vividly, and from almost that day on I started to avoid going in lifts if I possibly could. This continued right up into my twenties, by which time I only ever went in lifts if I absolutely had to. I had developed quite a significant phobia of lifts. So, what was my WCS? It was about getting stuck in a lift again, but actually it was more general than that – something about being in an enclosed space I couldn't get out of. And what was my reaction? To avoid going in lifts.

Of course, I started to avoid lifts because I wanted to avoid being that anxious – I was trying to make things better. And it seems the obvious thing to do: if something makes you anxious and you don't like being anxious, avoid that thing! The trouble is that as soon as I started to avoid lifts, something strange happened. You see, humans like to believe they are in control of the world around them. Once we start to avoid the feared thing, somehow our brain immediately starts to believe that we are personally stopping the WCS it is linked to from happening. I started to believe that the only reason I never got stuck in a lift was because I never went in one. The problem is that this also forms the belief that if you ever *don't* control that feared thing, the WCS *will* happen. So, as I quickly found out, avoiding lifts actually made me *more* scared of them. At first I just didn't like them but would go in if I had to. Pretty soon though, having to go in a lift filled me with terror. Even now, years after I have worked through my own phobia, I still start to sweat ever so slightly in that moment when the lift has stopped at the floor and the doors haven't started to open yet.

Growing anxiety

Anxiety is an emotion that quickly spreads like a forest fire, eating up more and more of our life without us realizing. Very often we find ourselves starting to avoid more and more things in a desperate attempt to control our fears. The things that trigger that anxiety can grow, meaning that it gradually affects more of our life. In my case, as my anxiety grew, I found that bit by bit other small spaces were starting to make me feel anxious and I started to feel the desire to avoid them too.

Here's another example of how anxiety can grow once we start to try to run away from it. A natural anxiety, and one that many people will admit to being a bit paranoid about, is having someone break into our car. So, when we leave the car, we are careful to lock it, which should decrease the anxiety. But one day, feeling a bit more anxious than usual (maybe it was a dodgy area, or maybe we had just had a hard day so were a bit more vulnerable to anxiety than usual), we find ourselves checking the driver's door is locked after we have pressed the magic button to lock it. Then, knowing it is definitely locked, we move on. Anxiety dealt with. We've all done it!

What anxiety does, however, is make us start to worry. From that moment on something somewhere inside us is not satisfied unless we check that driver's door every time we lock the car. Somewhere in our head we have started to believe that the WCS (having our car broken into) might happen if we do not complete that extra check. We never needed to check before but now somehow it feels as if we should and the anxiety doesn't go away until we do. Now, luckily for most of us, that is as far as it goes. But if for some reason we are more prone to anxiety than others, or if we are having a hard time and are generally very anxious (say, if we are under stress), we might find ourselves much more vulnerable to this anxiety. And one night, you absent-mindedly, barely aware of doing it, we check the boot as well. Suddenly we find that the anxiety only diminishes if we check both from that moment on – the door and the boot. Otherwise we cannot relax and enjoy whatever it is we are doing once we have left the car. Anxiety rarely stays still, and if we are not careful, it will win ground off us and gradually back us into a corner.

Anxiety like this can very easily tie us in knots. It can restrict our lives, and because the anxiety grows with every step we take to try to escape and run away from it, it can start to cause real problems. People with severe phobias find their life utterly controlled by them. Conditions can form, such as Obsessive Compulsive Disorder (OCD), in which people find themselves caught in beliefs that if they do not complete certain series of checks or actions, very serious worst case scenarios will happen. For people suffering from OCD, these rituals, designed in an attempt to keep anxiety at bay, often start to take over their life. So, as it increases, anxiety can make us much more prone to stress, and it can worsen a problem with stress that we already have.

Another key way in which anxiety can cause problems is if we actually fail to pick up that it is anxiety we are experiencing. Because anxiety is such a physical condition, all too often people can find that they mistake the physical symptoms for something else. So, anxiety is triggered and starts to cause physical symptoms such as increased heart rate or hyperventilating (taking lots of small shallow breaths). These things start to cause their own symptoms before long. We become aware of our heart racing even though we are not exercising. Then, as the fast breathing changes the chemistry of our blood (as the levels of oxygen and carbon dioxide change), that also causes symptoms such as dizziness, tingling in fingers or toes and even chest pain. If we did not realize that the trigger of these things was anxiety, this would be really frightening. We might start to worry that we were really ill, perhaps having a heart attack, or that we were going to pass out. Of course, that fear just makes the anxiety (and therefore the symptoms) worse. Pretty soon we are sweating too, wild-eyed and panicked. This is how a panic attack develops, and anyone who has ever had one or witnessed one will tell you just how 'physical' it looks and feels. It really does feel as if something is dreadfully physically wrong. But it is 'just' anxiety. I say 'just' because anxiety can be a very powerful and manipulative emotion, and the physical effects are real – they just aren't what you might think they are.

What makes some people more prone to anxiety than others?

Certain personality profiles make us more vulnerable to feeling anxious, perhaps because we build more rules and regulations into our lives (see Chapter 9 on personality). Or we might have had experiences in our childhood that make us more susceptible to anxiety as we try to avoid similar things happening again, or because that extreme stress experienced when we were young has actually affected our biological response to anxiety. Remember that emotions are triggered when our brains detect significant combinations of things going on around us. If, for whatever reason, our brain triggers more anxiety than most people's, we are more likely to end up reacting to it in that way that makes things worse.

Something else that affects how prone we are to anxiety problems is how well we tolerate the experience of anxiety. Some people do not mind feeling a bit anxious. In fact, they almost thrive on that experience of stress. They might describe themselves as 'adrenaline junkies' (adrenaline is one of the hormones released as part of anxiety that controls the whole physical experience it triggers) and love to do things where they are operating under pressure. Most people perform better with a little bit of anxiety because adrenaline helps us to concentrate and boosts our performance. But some people totally and utterly hate the experience of anxiety. This may be because they have had all too many experiences where it has built up and become overwhelming – perhaps in panic attacks or phobic reactions. They get to the stage where the slightest anxiety is terrifying and they will do anything to avoid feeling anxious. It's as if experiencing that first anxiety spark immediately triggers another because their brain links that feeling to something that has previously been a very bad experience. So, it triggers more anxiety... which triggers more anxiety... and so on. For these people anxiety builds up incredibly fast and becomes overwhelming, and many end up almost imprisoned in their own homes as they desperately try to avoid all the triggers for their anxiety.

So, if we are feeling trapped by our fears, what can we do about it?

The most effective treatment for any anxiety problem is to turn around and face it. Did you ever have a parent or sibling who used to chase you up the stairs when you were younger? Even though you knew who it was, it was somehow scary! Everything is more scary when we are running away from it, and anxiety is no different. If something makes us really scared, the best way to deal with it is to take back control and, instead of avoiding it, start to deliberately face up to it. Of course, if you have a severe phobia or struggle with really intense fear, you will need some help with this and it is possible to be referred to a psychologist or CBT (Cognitive Behavioural Therapy) specialist who can help you to work through your fears and win some of that ground back bit by bit.

The point of facing your fears is to start to retrain your brain. We need to teach it that actually, even if we are exposed to that so feared thing, the worst case scenario doesn't necessarily happen. We gradually need to build up experiences in which we do expose ourselves to that feared stimulus without anything bad actually happening. Bit by bit our brain will start to learn that it simply doesn't need to trigger that extreme fear reaction every time we are in that position.

Of course, treatment doesn't usually make you face your worst fears straight away, and if you are trying to work things out on your own, it's important that you don't jump right in with the thing that terrifies you most. It's about working out the most sensible step you can take without risking trying to jump too far and failing – because that can make the fear feel stronger. Most therapists will ask you to make a list of the things that would trigger your fear, starting with the most scary and working backwards. So, to return to the example of my own lift phobia, the worst thing would have been going in one of those scary car-park lifts that look really scary and have no windows (you know, the big metal ones). Working back from there, I could make a list of things that got a bit easier with each step. Lifts in busy areas are less scary, as are those with big windows. Lifts with just a few people in are not too bad, but cramming people in like sardines makes any lift worse. You keep making this list until you have got down to the smallest step that you can think of that relates to your fear. When I started to tackle my lift phobia, the first thing I would do was stand and watch people going in and out of lifts and just note in my head that none of them got stuck. It was a small step but it started me winning ground back off the anxiety. Gradually I was able to start to go in lifts myself (the non-scary ones at first!), and bit by bit the anxiety started to go down.

Winning ground back from anxiety can take time but it is worth it! If you are aware that anxiety is starting to take over your life, do go and talk it through with your doctor. They may be able to refer you for some treatment to help you to start winning ground back.

9 Personality and stress

I wonder if, as you have been reading this book so far, you have identified with the kinds of signs, symptoms and experiences that have been mentioned where stress is concerned. Issues with stress are obviously more common if you go and talk to people who work in very stressful jobs, or people who pack in a lot around the edges of their job – parents who juggle work and childcare, or people who work full-time but also do voluntary work in their 'free' time. But the truth is that people vary in how much stress affects them. You may know someone who works with you, or a friend or family member, who seems immune to stress. They appear to be able to work under immense pressure, to juggle many demands and responsibilities at once, to take tests and challenges on their shoulders without the slightest struggle. They manage all these things and still seem unruffled, perfectly calm and together. We all know people like this – and we love to hate them! Why can't we manage that same degree of cool efficiency? Of course, one possibility is that it is all an illusion and they are just very good at bluffing (we hope!), but it remains true that some people are just less affected by stress than others.

Meanwhile, others (you may place yourself in this category) find themselves struggling with stress much more than many around them. They find themselves utterly frustrated as they realize the impact stress is having on them, and often feel a total failure when stress forces them to scale back what they do. Some are forced to give up jobs they love or things they really long to do, simply because they find that stress has too big an impact on them, on their family life or on their health. So, what is it that makes one person so much more prone to damaging stress than another?

At the root of some of this variation is personality – the way our minds are made up, the things that make all of us think and react in different ways. Personality factors, which often pass down families, very strongly influence things such as the way we think about and see the world around us, as well as have a role to play in the development of our own identity – what we think about *ourselves*. The interesting thing about personality is that all personality features have a good and a bad side. For example, you might get someone who prides themselves on how reliable and precise they are. This is a great thing in some careers and probably something they would say is one of their good qualities, but someone working alongside them might talk of how impatient they were, how they were not very good at delegating tasks because they felt they always did them better themselves. The same personality can look good – or bad – depending on the perspective you take!

So, how does personality relate to stress?

Remember that there are different kinds of trigger for stress. On the one hand, stress is caused by the genuine physical demand that certain tasks place on our bodies. If we are trying to work hard for a long period of time, there is a physical need to concentrate and focus on what we are doing. However, much of our modern-day, twenty-first-century stress is caused by social and emotional triggers. These are things such as emotions, triggered when our brain detects something we might need to respond to, or social situations (often linked with those emotions) in which we have to react and interact. Although personality cannot change the physical triggers of stress, it is a bit like the filter through which our brain sees the world. So, although personality can't change, for example, how much attention is required to drive a car for four hours, it can affect how we respond to incidents that might happen on that drive. Personality can also influence how likely we are to put ourselves in situations that will prove to be stressful. Personality can take the base level of stress *anyone* would have experienced and add to it.

It might not be surprising, therefore, that certain personality traits seem to be more prone to problems with stress than others. Perhaps you have heard about Type A personality? People like this are very competitive and impatient. They push themselves very hard and often expect the same high standards of others around them. They are typically very intelligent and willing to put in hard work to get results. They love to work in high-adrenaline environments and often pursue leisure pursuits outside of work that are just as high-adrenaline. Sound like anyone you know? Type A personality has been linked with a statistically higher risk of many of the physical consequences of stress, such as cardiovascular problems.

Perfectionism

Probably the most common personality trait linked with stress is that of perfectionism. In fact, perfectionism is something linked with a lot of negative health outcomes – mental and physical. Perfectionism is a complicated personality type, which can be expressed in various different ways. On the whole though, people who are perfectionists push themselves very hard and can be single-minded in their pursuit of the things they are aiming for. They set themselves high goals and are often very hard on themselves. What is interesting about perfectionism is the way that it is linked in research both with high achievement (many successful sports stars score highly on charts of perfectionism, as do high achievers in other areas such as business) and with various mental and physical health problems. It's clear that something about personality features like this can be both very positive but, at the same time, very negative. Perfectionism is linked not just to stress but also to an increased risk of many emotional and psychological problems. Some experts have even called for it to be declared an illness in its own right!

So, what is it about certain mindsets that can sometimes cause people to start to struggle when they are under stress? In fact, it is research into the personality trait of perfectionism that gives us a chance to understand better the issue of personality. Studies into perfectionism in people who have become unwell often look at those with eating disorders such as anorexia. The personality trait of perfectionism is hugely more common in those with anorexia than the general public. These studies look at the ways in which people 'show' their perfectionism before and after treatment. What this research is interested in is whether recovery from anorexia includes 'getting rid' of perfectionism or not, telling us something very important about the impact that character trait can have. In fact, what they show is that recovered sufferers tend to continue to score highly on measures of perfectionism; however, the way that perfectionism is expressed has changed – and something about that seems to have taken the sting out of it and stopped it having such a damaging effect. This message is really important as it shows us that managing stress more effectively isn't about trying to change the people we were made to be. What it does mean, though, is that something about our personality might carry with it a potential weakness that makes us more vulnerable to stress – and that we can change.

What is it that can make some personalities so risky in times of stress? Again and again, two issues are shown to be significant. The key is not simply whether we are a perfectionist, or a Type A personality, or anything else; the key is something to do with what those kinds of mindsets might lead us to do in order to compensate for something else we struggle with. Research shows that we are most likely to start to have problems if we use aspects of our personality for one of two things: either to cope with anxiety or as something we build our self-esteem on.

Let's look at those two things in a bit more detail. Anxiety, as we've seen in the previous chapter, is a hugely common problem and one that tends to be exacerbated by stress. Stress stimulates the release of adrenaline, which makes us feel even more anxious, and very soon it can become a vicious cycle. Often it is tempting to deal with anxiety by trying to do things to help us to feel in control of the things we are anxious about. We looked at the example of checking that the car is locked in order to get rid of the worry that it might be broken into. That checking behaviour makes us feel more in control – we start to think, 'Because I have checked, it won't get broken into' – and that is why it makes us less anxious.

Now, if you are a perfectionist, you are already more likely to have a basic belief that you should always do things to a very high standard. People who score highly on measures of perfectionism are often the kinds of people who will write themselves lists, check things off or have mental checklists of things they feel they need to do. It's not a great leap to a place where you start to slip into using this natural tendency, which you are very at home with, to try to control anxiety. If stress at work or at home is starting to trigger a lot of anxiety, you might find yourself more and more having to check that you have done certain things properly. Visual things such as tidiness or orderliness might start to become more important. You might find your brain running anxiously through checklists of things you need to do and emails you have to send, tasks you have to do and people you need to see. Some people might transfer their stress to other areas and start to push themselves very hard, perhaps in some kind of sport, constantly trying to improve their personal best or always having to achieve a certain level or standard.

Behind this is a sense that if we manage to do these things, the source of the anxiety will go away and the WCS, whatever it is (although exactly what it is you are anxious about may be very vague if you are just generally stressed), will not happen. Sometimes it is a more general goal that is used to control anxiety. So, we might feel fine as long as we are achieving at a very high standard but start to dread making an error and being proved imperfect. We expect the best and push ourselves very hard because we know that if we don't, that fear might become overwhelming. That is how people with a personality that makes them prone to perfectionism can easily get caught in using it to control anxiety. Thinking in that way is linked to a whole host of problems, from eating disorders to workaholism, as they struggle to try to control everything in their life.

Self-esteem

The second common way these personalities can cause problems is if we build our self-esteem upon them. Self-esteem is an interesting and significant phenomenon, which we'll explore in much more detail later. It's about that vital issue of what we think about *ourselves*, and it is very important to have 'good enough' self-esteem in life. We don't have to think we are amazing, but we do need to think enough of ourselves. Without 'good enough' self-esteem, people simply don't try anything because they don't have the belief in themselves to think they might be able to achieve it. This becomes another vicious cycle, then, as they see themselves as worthless and failures because they never try: they never get the chance to build up their self-esteem. If we are someone who is very intelligent and tends to achieve very highly, we can easily see how our self-esteem might become based around that. So we grow up with a belief that we are valuable *because* we are good at things. After all, self-esteem is built from the messages about themselves that children get back from adults around them, so if the message is constantly related to how well they have achieved, it is easy to get the message that they are valuable *because they achieve well*. Fast-forward that child on twenty or so years and we have someone working in a high-achieving, hard-fought world; someone who cannot take their foot off the accelerator because ultimately, when it comes down to it, achieving is *who they are*. Without what they do, they are nothing; they are not sure why they would have a purpose or a value. We all get some of our self-esteem from what we do and achieve, but this is someone whose whole world is built on that basis. Theories about the root of Type A personality suggest that it describes someone using perfectionist tendencies to try to make up for or disguise a problem with low self-esteem. This is someone who is using a tendency they already had to push themselves hard and achieve very highly in order to try to stop themselves feeling insecure. Someone who does this runs a much greater risk of stress having a negative impact on their life.

Ultimately, both of these tendencies are risky because they place so much weight on something that just isn't possible. They both lead us to make rules or goals in our mind that are very hard to live up to. So we say, 'I must always get things right,' or 'Everyone must always like me for me to be acceptable.' And that's the key to why stress tends to end up having an emotional impact: it leads us to attempt solutions that simply are not going to work in the long term. No matter how hard we try, no human can ever manage to be totally perfect. But many of us have found ourselves under tremendous pressure to be just that, living with a belief that we must continue to achieve the near impossible. Every time we fail our brain triggers more emotion, and we put ourselves under renewed pressure to try to get it right. This means that many of us go through life as humans trying to be super-people. We might keep it up for a while, maybe even for a long time. With enough work, enough brains and some good luck, we can manage to maintain the illusion of perfection for a while, but it will take its toll. And that is when, if we have so much resting on it, we may start to find that some basic things about our world and what we think about ourselves will start to crumble. Trying to be a super-person is exhausting and very stressful, because at any moment our cover could be blown and it might become apparent that we are... just human.

How do we know if we have a personality that might be making us more susceptible to stress?

One clue might be in the kinds of thoughts that we are prone to. There's more about those in Chapter 10, but if aspects of our personality are putting us under pressure, it is probably apparent in the way we think. This is likely to be a more reliable measure than just whether we think we are a perfectionist or not. In my experience, I have found that a lot of people who put themselves under pressure because of this tendency in their personality really resist any suggestion that they are a perfectionist because they think they are nowhere near good enough to be perfect! Or they will proudly point out the total chaos and mess on their desk and claim this is proof that they cannot be a perfectionist. But there is more than one way in which this kind of personality is expressed, so do not fall into the trap of the stereotypes you might read about. In fact, if I look from day to day at the kind of behaviour that is triggering stress for people I work with, it is often subtle things that are causing the problem. It isn't aiming to be *perfect*, more just pushing ourselves to do that little bit more than most people would. So it isn't good enough to just do something well enough; we want to do it *really* well. It isn't just getting the kids off to school on time; it is making sure that they never forget anything and are all immaculately dressed, with their hair done and everything looking lovely. It isn't just making sure those friends we invite round have a nice evening; it is trying to make it *really* good, cooking all the food ourselves, tidying frantically so the house is beautiful, remembering to buy candles for the dinner table... (Note that this last one can often masquerade as us being terribly caring about those other people and wanting to do it for them – we need to watch out for perfectionism expressed as wanting our relationships with other people to be perfect!) It isn't just getting ourselves out of the door on time; it is that little thought that says, 'If I really rush, I could get the washing on before I go out.' Those little subtle things can be the way that perfectionism, or a tendency to push ourselves hard, can gradually add to our stress and leave us starting to struggle.

Personality cannot on its own create a problem with stress. And even if your own personality has a role to play in why you do struggle with stress, it's important not to throw out the baby with the bathwater. Remember, your personality might mean you are more vulnerable to stress problems, but the same personality also means you have that great potential. So, if you have recognized something of yourself in this chapter, the same things can actually be very positive characteristics: that urge to push yourself to achieve just that little bit more – that fuels little things but also means that you are probably very driven in what you do. Don't feel down about yourself because of who you are. We all need to learn to be aware of the potential weaknesses of our personality – our Achilles heel – which might mean that our personality causes us some problems. This is not about needing to change your personality – not about trying to be someone you are not. In fact, it is about releasing you from the impact of stress so that you have more chance of being everything you were made to be. Remember, you were made unique as the person you are – so be aware of the potential weak points that your personality gives you where stress is concerned, but go out and be that person the best you can be.

10 I think, therefore I am! Thinking styles, stress and creating emotional bonfires

The last few chapters have taken us on a journey of understanding the ways in which our emotions and personality can be part of a problem with stress. We've looked at what emotions are and what they are designed to do, and how they act like sparks to trigger our attention and help us analyse things going on around us that may or may not be significant. We've also understood how certain patterns of thinking or types of personality can result in something that works like kindling – thoughts and beliefs which can catch fire when an emotion spark is triggered and result in an emotional blaze. What all of this has shown us again and again is that there are two ways in which specific things about our thinking and beliefs can leave us prone to having lots of difficult emotions to deal with.

Challenges to our world view

The first occurs if we have in our minds certain goals, rules or ideas which we try to live by, but which are very often challenged by the world around us: beliefs that we have about ourselves or others, or simply as a result of the natural uncertainty that life often throws at us. These can be things we have learned in childhood or things that other people have taught us about ourselves or the world. As children we have no idea how the world works, so as we grow we start to put together these beliefs and rules which help us to understand better – rather like the brain's basic 'how to' manual for the world at large! On the whole, problems occur when we learn a rule or belief as a child that either simply isn't true for the adult world or ceases to be helpful once we are adults.

So, let's say that as a child we were taught that life is basically fair – good things happen to good people and we make our own luck. This has become one of the rules we expect the world to fit in with. In reality, of course, life isn't always like that, so we might find that as an adult this belief is challenged frequently as unfortunate circumstances, bad luck and really difficult and painful things happen to the people we love and care for. So, our best friend loses his job, a colleague struggles with bad health, or even smaller difficulties we are having – all these things are experiences that clash with a basic idea we have of how the world *should* work. Those people seem like good people to us, and we try to be good ourselves, but bad things keep happening. Each time that clash is identified by our brain, an emotion will be triggered.

What about another example? A few years ago I worked with a woman called Christine, who had grown up with very highly achieving parents. She was the eldest of three children, and to most people looking at her she had been pretty successful in her life. She had a good job in a big company, a nice house and was married with two children.

However, Christine could never shake the thought that she wasn't good enough. Even in work situations in which her colleagues thought she was the most skilled for the job, she felt unsure and worried a lot about underperforming. She admitted to having a dreadful fear of failure that haunted her and she used to lie awake at night worrying about what people would think about her. She had come to me because she was struggling with stress and felt she was near a breakdown. She was starting to have to take time off work and was struggling with some medical problems.

For Christine, one of the most significant things we did was work on understanding why she was experiencing so much stress. She had grown up in a family where the most important thing was not just to achieve but to be outstanding – one of the best, if not *the* best, at whatever she did. Her parents had put a lot of pressure on her and she had been to a school where success was everything. Even though she had done well, it simply hadn't been enough in her parents' eyes; they always seemed disappointed with her eventual career and criticized her openly for all kinds of aspects of her life. Christine admitted that she pushed herself very hard and that she never allowed herself to stop or take a break, even if she was exhausted. Christine had grown up with the rule that she must always do everything she could to achieve extremely highly. Indeed, she had learned from her parents and her school that if she didn't, then she wasn't worthwhile as a person. Now in her adult life this belief was triggering an avalanche of anxiety as she worried about failing or felt that her achievements might not be good enough.

One final example. One thing about children is that on the whole they like life to be predictable. Children have a basic belief that everything happens for a reason – simple cause and effect. But for some, life is actually very out of control or unpredictable, perhaps because their living circumstances change a lot or because someone significant in their life is struggling and emotionally volatile. In those circumstances children often take responsibility themselves for the emotions and reactions of someone else, even though they are nothing to do with them. It's less scary to a child to do that than to admit that actually the world is not a safe, predictable place. So, a child with a parent who can be violent will desperately try to understand what they are doing to trigger it. As a result, they often grow up believing that they should be able to keep other people around them happy all the time. They are often very good at picking up on other people's emotions because in their childhood they had to be in order to try to avoid frightening or even dangerous situations. But imagine how they would feel if a person they care about is experiencing something that is making them miserable but that no one else can change. To someone who believes they can and should be able to keep everyone around them happy, a situation like this is very hard and will trigger some difficult feelings. They might try all kinds of things to attempt to help and exhaust themselves or annoy others in the process. It isn't easy to accept that some things in the world are just not the way that they learned they would be.

I like to call emotions triggered in this way 'echo emotions'. It's as if we have the emotion itself – the emotion anyone would have experienced in that situation – but we also have the echo of something else – the memories that caused the rule or goal we carry with us as part of who we are. If something around us contradicts that rule, risks that goal or challenges that belief, we will have an emotional reaction. Of course, more often than not we are completely unaware of these rules and goals that we live life by. This means that the emotions they trigger can feel out of our control or illogical. We might worry that we are reacting irrationally but, without an understanding of where these feelings are coming from, we are powerless to deal with them. The emotions can also be very powerful, especially if they are linked to very painful memories or traumatic episodes that happened in our past. Of course, the more of these kind of rules and beliefs we have, the more emotions we will find triggered day to day that we have to deal with – and that can leave us very vulnerable to stress.

Emotional kindling

As we have already learned, the second thing that can leave us vulnerable by triggering these negative emotions is if there is kindling around in our minds that can be ignited by those emotion sparks when they occur and go on to create emotional fires. So, what exactly is thought 'kindling'? Research has shown that there are certain kinds of thoughts that can be very unhelpful in that they can make emotions 'grow' and become more powerful. These kinds of thoughts are generally not based on fact and may be more likely in people who have certain personalities or certain beliefs about the world around them or about themselves. Read the following examples and see if any sound familiar to you.

Negative styles of thinking: These are thinking styles that would be held by the classic pessimist! They are about focusing on the negative things that have happened, while ignoring anything positive; they predict negative things in the future no matter what; they play down any success

103

but play up any failure. So, someone might find themselves thinking, 'What a dreadful day,' concentrating on one or two things that happened that were not so great but ignoring the many good things they did achieve. They might worry about things that are likely to happen in the future, predicting negative outcomes: 'I bet that meeting tomorrow will be a total disaster too.' Even when they do well, they will play it down: 'I think my boss must have been feeling sorry for me'; whereas if things go badly, they take all the blame: 'I was totally useless today, I'm such a disaster, I never get anything right!'

All-or-nothing thinking: This pattern of thinking is very common, both in teenagers and young people who tend to see the world in more of a black and white way, and in adults who are prone to perfectionist-style thinking. All-or-nothing thinking describes someone who tends to think of things as either one thing or the other with no grey areas between. Something is either good enough or it is not; it is either right or wrong. People who think in this way tend to set very high standards and do not allow for any margins when they – or other people – are working towards those aims. So, if they write a report and feel that they have not done it to their usual very high standard, it is a total failure, even if it is still very good. Sometimes people with this tendency will actively look for signs of failure and then declare their work useless and feel totally dissatisfied with the outcome. They may also apply this strict rule to social occasions, feeling, for example, that an evening they have planned was a total disaster just because one person was suddenly unable to come at the last minute or because one small thing didn't go according to their precise plan. This style of thinking can combine with catastrophizing (see below) to lead people to feel extremes of emotion when things do not go 100 per cent well for them. It should be noted that it can also cause problems in relationships because working for, or being in a relationship with, someone who expects these kind of exacting standards can be very challenging. You can spot someone who is prone to this kind of thinking by their use of a lot of words such as 'should' or 'ought to'. They might say or think things such as 'I *should* be able to get this done' or 'I *ought to* make sure I get that right', and they often struggle with a lot of guilt when they fail to meet the high standard they push themselves to achieve.

Catastrophizing: This refers to a pattern of thinking that tends to happen when we are under stress, anxious or worried about something. Sometimes called snowballing, it describes the way in which our mind can make great illogical jumps between something that has happened now (or we fear may happen) and things that may or may not be true or may happen in the future. So, we might accidentally say the wrong thing to a colleague. This leaves us feeling bad and triggers thoughts such as 'Oh no, they will tell everyone I was horrible to them'. This then leads us to start worrying – 'Everyone will think I am a horrid person... no one will like me... no one will want to know me' – and before we know it we have moved on to worrying about future things –'I will always be alone... I'll never get married... I'll die all alone!' Although reading a typical thread of catastrophizing thoughts may seem almost comical, in the moment it feels as bad as that last thought – as if something we did inadvertently, a throw away remark to a colleague, may have sealed our fate for life that we will live and die alone. Catastrophizing triggers strong feelings such as anxiety and fear, as well as hopelessness and depression as we feel that there is nothing we can do to stop these dreadful things coming true.

Emotional reasoning: We've looked at how important emotions are, acting a bit like smoke alarms, warning us of possible issues we need to pay attention to. But sometimes we make a basic mistake about what we think emotions are. Rather than understanding that they warn us of possible problems, we assume they mean actual problems! So, if we feel anxious, we feel the thing we are dreading really *will* happen. Or we feel guilty and therefore assume we *are* guilty. This is like hearing a smoke alarm and assuming it always means there is a fire, when, in fact, everyone knows it usually just means the toast is done! It is a very common problem where negative emotions are concerned.

Personalization: This is an interesting one because it is a very common tendency but one that also has an obvious positive side to it. This describes someone who tends to take responsibility for things – things that may not even be anything to do with them. They are great people to have around because we can really rely on them, but it also means they are prone to feeling very guilty about things that just weren't their fault at all. They might feel very guilty or upset because someone else struggles to make any friends at a social event, or feel bad if something wasn't done, even if it wasn't their job to do it in the first place. They are the person who felt guilty at school if the class was told off, even if they had never done the thing they were being told off for! They find it hard to know where their responsibility ends and someone else's begins, and may be prone to running around other people who might take advantage of this apparently very caring side to their nature. Spot this thinking pattern by thoughts such as 'I should have done that' or 'I wish I had known she felt like that', or the constant feelings of guilt.

Negative mind reading: This last common unhelpful thinking pattern describes someone who would probably describe themselves as being very good at 'reading' people. And to some degree it is true, for they certainly spend a lot of time reacting to things that they have 'picked up' from other people. The trouble is that they tend only to pick up on negative things they think others are thinking, and they may not always be very accurate. This thinking style often occurs in someone who is struggling with feeling quite insecure and is not very confident about themselves, particularly in social situations. They feel very anxious about what others are thinking and sometimes project their worst fears on to people without any actual evidence to support their conclusions. They might think, 'Those people are laughing at me,' or 'Well, he obviously doesn't want to talk to me,' or 'She thinks I am a real idiot,' without any real reason to think this. Something as simple as people laughing when they enter a room, or stopping talking when they walk by, can be enough to push them into a cycle of worrying about what those people were thinking of them. This thinking style can be a real problem because it ultimately pushes people into isolation as they start to avoid the social situations that trigger these kind of thoughts and feelings.

Do you recognize any of these tendencies yourself? Well, I would be surprised if you didn't, because all of us think in some of these ways sometimes, particularly on a bad day or if we are stressed. And the chances are that most of us also carry some of those rules or beliefs that can also cause problems. On the whole, those things do not cause any serious problems. However, when we are under stress, it is as if someone turns the heat up underneath our thought patterns, and sometimes under that extra pressure they can then start to cause problems. If you have started to have some emotional problems – related to stress or not – the chances are that some of these patterns of thinking are making things worse. Tending to think in these ways is like having a mind full of kindling, so that negative emotions catch fire, last longer and grow.

What can you do about it?

So, what do you do if this does describe you and you know, or suspect, that the way you think or the things you believe about the world are part of your problem with stress? The first step is to spend some time understanding better why you react the way you do. This may involve identifying unhelpful thinking patterns, or even starting to understand some of the underlying beliefs and goals that might be affecting you. Now, you might wonder how this can help – surely it is not changing anything? But the truth is that once you understand why you react in a certain way, you also inherently become aware of the option of doing something different. Without understanding, you are just reacting instinctively and automatically. Understanding is the first step towards being able to make changes. It's a bit like those old computer games where we had to work our way across a giant world, solving puzzles and finding objects. Often in those games there were whole areas of the 'world' that we couldn't get to unless we were holding the right object or had found a certain key. If we did have the right thing in the right place at the right time, suddenly doors opened or new bits of screen magically appeared! In a similar way, once we become aware that something inside us makes us react a certain way, we also suddenly see other options – alternative ways to react, different actions we could take instead. Another analogy is to think of the way our mind normally works as doing a dance. We have learned certain steps to the dance and we automatically dance them without thinking. Only when we become aware of the steps we are taking can we then start to think about learning a different dance – perhaps one that leaves us less prone to stress or experiencing fewer difficult emotions.

In fact, looking in more detail at these kinds of thing is what Cognitive Behavioural Therapy (CBT) does – something you may have heard about as it is becoming a very popular form of psychological treatment for many different illnesses. CBT explores the way in which thinking patterns can affect the way we feel, act and react, and looks at the beliefs that underlie them. We'll take a look at some of the approaches that CBT uses in Chapter 14, but if you think that you might benefit from a course of CBT, do talk to your doctor. Another option, and one open to almost everyone, is to look at one of the free websites that take you through a course of CBT, examining your tendency to think in certain ways and helping you to challenge that.[1]

Often when we are looking at problems with stress, we look outside of ourselves and blame or try to change the situations we are in. This chapter has looked at some of the ways in which we might be our own worst enemy, thinking and reacting in ways that are not actually helpful and might worsen our vulnerability to stress, so that we struggle to cope where others may not be affected. If reading this has made you determined to look at the way you think and make some changes, remember that it does take time! You have spent all of your life so far learning to think this way, so give yourself time to change it. You might find too that you do need some support, particularly if the reason you have certain rules or put certain pressure on yourself comes from something in your past. Challenging what are often automatic thoughts is not easy, so get some help. Remember also that sometimes that pressure comes from things outside of you – a difficult boss with very high expectations, or a job where you are asked to do things you are just not capable of or don't have the time or necessary authority to do. If that is the situation, don't take all the blame yourself. Do look at your thinking, but also think about how you can make some changes to the situation that is placing you under so much unnecessary pressure.

11 Self-esteem: knowing who you are

Before we move on from looking at things that can make us more vulnerable to stress, we need to take a more detailed look at self-esteem. Self-esteem is something that you will have heard mentioned many times. Over the last decade it has become one of the most often discussed psychological issues, as research looks into its impact on issues as far separated as family life and violent crime. Self-esteem seems to be a very important part of who we are as human beings. But what exactly is it, where does it come from, and how does *your* self-esteem have an influence on how you respond to stress?

As you would expect for such a widely discussed and debated phenomenon, there are various definitions of self-esteem. In essence though, self-esteem is a measure of the person we think we are, of what we feel our value is, and something to do with what we understand about our place in the world. Self-esteem affects the way we act and react to things, and our confidence and belief in ourselves, as well as practical things such as how successful we are likely to be in both work/academic achievement and in relationships and social challenges. Some people would separate the concepts of self-esteem (how valuable or worthy we feel we are) and self-identity or self-image (the detail of *who* we think we are). However, I am deliberately going to merge them because, in a practical sense of the way they influence us, they very much overlap.

Self-esteem in childhood

The roots of self-esteem are developed in our early childhood. In fact, that is one of the most fascinating things about self-esteem because something that can have such a huge impact on our adult life is actually developed in the years that, as adults, we may have little or no memory of. When a child is very young, they have no idea of who they are. At first they do not even understand that they are separate from their mother or main caregiver. As they get older and start to understand this, their concept of themselves as a separate person starts to develop. Alongside this, their brain gradually matures and they start to gain the ability to form what will later (much later!) become their adult self-esteem.

So, our self-esteem developed when we were very young. In fact, studies suggest that for most people our self-esteem at age four or five is a pretty good indicator of our adult self-esteem. At this age we are hugely dependent on the significant people around us to help build our self-esteem. Children are like a blank canvas, with no idea of who they are, what they are good at or what their character is like. So, when adults comment on things ('You're *really* good at that, well done!') or when children hear things said about themselves ('Amy is very good at getting on with other children'), all of those statements and snippets of information are gathered together and start to form that very naive self-esteem. Much has been made, therefore, of the importance of praising young children and giving them lots of good and positive feedback. Actually, however, the most important thing is that we get both a positive and also a reasonably accurate idea of who we are. Children also get feedback from how they perform in various skills, and parental comments, no matter how enthusiastic, will not cancel out the fact that a child knows that they are not very good at something. This is particularly the case for very intelligent children, who tend to be quite hard on themselves if they feel they have not performed well. One teenager I worked with recalled becoming suspicious at a very early age of her mother's always effusive praise: 'She always said everything I did was amazing, and I started to get suspicious. So one day I drew something really useless, deliberately. It was just like a line on a piece of paper. I took it to her to see what she thought and she said it was brilliant and put it on the fridge. I never really believed the things she said again after that.'

One thing at this age that can be very powerful is the impact of labels on small children. Because they are such sponges for information about themselves, and because the only source of information they have is the people around them, they can be very vulnerable to labels or comments that are made. They will even start to act in a way that fits with those labels. So, the child who is always reported to be 'the quiet one' learns quickly that being 'quiet' is part of who they are. Instinctively, then, on some level they start to act in a way that fits with that – because being quiet is something they have learned about who they are. Labels can come from all kinds of places, but often stem from where we were in the family we grew up in. If we have an elder brother or sister who was always quite demanding, we may have been the second child who was always 'so much easier and well behaved'. Or, the opposite may be true: we may be the child who was 'always a nightmare, never sat still'! These labels can be very powerful, particularly if they are negative, and it can be interesting to think back (or to question our parents!) and find out what sort of child we were. One person I worked with in their adult life had never really got over going to the same school as her older siblings and enduring several years of hearing

'She isn't as bright as her sisters'. Labels at this age can be very powerful because they are so readily taken on board as part of that self-identity. So, if they are used a lot and taken on board by the family, or by other prominent adults, they can then go on to become a self-fulfilling prophecy. The child who is a 'nightmare' continues to be one and is a behavioural challenge both at home and at school, whereas the child who is always 'as good as gold' always conforms, perhaps too much, never really feeling they can be themselves and express what they feel. Even apparently jokey labels – throwaway comments or family jokes – can be surprisingly powerful for children who are learning every day about who they are. Comments that we were the 'unplanned child' or that our dad 'was really hoping for a girl/boy', if repeated consistently throughout a childhood, can easily become part of our self-concept.

Once the naive basis of self-esteem has formed, it tends to be fairly stable throughout childhood, and, in the most part, fairly positive. Children have a baseline self-esteem that is generally positive, and even in the situations where there are some negative seeds planted, or where life is very traumatic, they have a remarkable resilience. But this is the foundation of adult self-esteem, and if there are weaknesses there, often they do not become apparent and develop further until the next time self-esteem is challenged. This happens during adolescence as part of the barrage of changes that comes once we hit puberty.

Self-esteem in adolescence

It used to be thought that the brain only dramatically changed and developed during early childhood, but with the advent of technology such as PET scanners and MRI we have been able to understand a lot more about the way the brain develops. Now scientists have shown that in adolescence the brain changes almost as much as in toddlerhood. The changes are in a different region though, and just as toddlers are tentatively, hesitantly and sometimes not very successfully learning basic skills such as speech and how to walk, run and hop, teenagers are learning the adult skills linked with things such as emotion (particularly more complex social emotions such as jealousy and love), motivation and, of course, self-esteem. As the teenage brain develops, adolescents start to acquire an abstract concept of who they are. Details such as what they are and are not good at, what they look like and how other people react to them become very important.

Children are very egocentric – that is, they genuinely believe the world revolves around them. This is one of the reasons why children struggle to appreciate that significant changes in their life, such as parents getting divorced, are not their fault, because to a child everything that happens is in some way connected to them. Teenagers start to realize that other people have a whole different perspective on the world, and as part of this their self-esteem starts to be influenced by much more than just what their parents think. Their friends and peers become crucial as they start to compare themselves to the people around them. In essence, they are asking themselves the question 'Am I normal?' and their self-esteem development can be profoundly affected by the results of this comparison. This is why it is so important for teenagers to wear the right clothes, have the right gadgets; even why it is so crucial that their parents are the same as other parents and don't do anything too embarrassingly different.

The other thing that affects teenagers' self-esteem is the

second abstract concept they form in their brains. Alongside what they think of themselves, they also start to think about what others think of them – and therefore what they think they *should* be like. This is influenced by many things – for example, the media (studies show that teenagers are the most susceptible to images in the media of very slim or beautiful models, and the most likely to feel bad about themselves as a result of those images) or parental or teacher expectations (so being the student most likely to get straight As can be a difficult pressure to bear). They are also influenced by their own personality. Teenagers who are more prone to perfectionism tend to put more pressure on themselves and are more likely to set very high standards (which, being human, they probably won't meet) or be very hard on themselves if they do feel they have 'failed'.

We can start to see now where problems with self-esteem can come from. Teenage development is when the final touches to adult self-esteem occur – the house built on the foundation laid in childhood. So, things that affect our self-esteem as teenagers really are important. Most teenagers (particularly girls) go through a dip in their self-esteem in the adolescent years – not surprising given the scrutiny and pressure they endure. But for some, that low self-esteem never resolves and they go into adult life struggling with who they think they are. Issues that date as far back as early childhood can start to become a problem as we try to build an adult self-esteem on a foundation that just cannot carry the weight. Or some of the classic experiences that so many of us endure as adolescents can genuinely challenge our concept of ourselves. Being very different to others, not fitting in at home or at school, being bullied or being the odd one out, struggling under the pressure of a parent who sets very high

116

goals and is never satisfied, a teacher who constantly criticizes, or a home life that is generally chaotic and non-supportive – all these things can be really difficult for teenagers trying to put together an adult self-concept.

Self-esteem in adulthood

As adults, what we all hope for is that we carry with us what I call 'good enough' self-esteem. Low self-esteem is an obvious problem, but sometimes having too high a self-esteem can also be an issue. Many of the people I work with worry terribly about becoming arrogant or selfish if they think too much of themselves. But actually thinking *enough* of ourselves is terribly important, and if we do not, it can trigger problems such as negative emotions or make us more prone to some of the unhelpful thinking patterns outlined in Chapter 10.

Figure 9: The six sources of adult self-esteem

1. Our concept of whether we are a basically good person or not

2. The opinions and support of those closest to us and whose opinion matters the most to us (family – and for those who have a faith, God)

3. Our academic ability (how clever we think we are)

4. What we think of our appearance

5. Feedback from others (including people such as our boss, colleagues, or friends – do they approve of us or not?)

6. How successful we are (how we perform in comparison to others in all kinds of areas such as competitions, exams, life...)

So, what about your self-esteem *now*? As adults we tend to get our self-esteem from roughly six areas, which you can see in figure 9. In a way, we can visualize our adult self-esteem as a pie chart, with each of these things giving more or less to the 'pie' (see figure 10). Most of us have a reasonably good balance; we get our self-esteem from a selection of these things – some more, some less, with some variation throughout our life. Remember, the ability to successfully build that 'pie' depends on what happens to you as a child and as a teenager.

Figure 10: One example of adult self-esteem balance

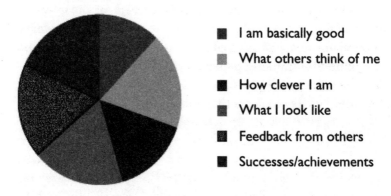

- I am basically good
- What others think of me
- How clever I am
- What I look like
- Feedback from others
- Successes/achievements

Where do problems with self-esteem come from and how can we recognize them?

If we think of that self-esteem 'pie', there are basically four things that commonly go wrong or cause us problems as adults. The first, and perhaps most common, is the question of whether, as teenagers, we have a foundation that gives us **'good enough' self-esteem**. If that foundation is strong enough, that teenager is likely to be reasonably confident and happy and be able to weather the many challenges of adolescence successfully. This gives them the opportunity and necessary confidence to build up further self-esteem, as they have the belief in themselves to try new things, take some measured risks, and generally learn more about who they are and what they can do. In contrast, the teenager with a poor foundation often struggles; they will already have doubts about who they are and difficult labels and beliefs about themselves restricting who they can be. They encounter problems with relationships, in school and elsewhere, and may withdraw or give up completely. Often even outstanding ability in one area such as academic work is not enough to counteract this gulf in self-esteem, and even very able young people can struggle as they try to understand why they have any value – often to the confusion of those around them who think they are totally brilliant. Low self-esteem like this can be all-encompassing and affect every area of life. It affects our thinking styles, making the unhelpful patterns in Chapter 10 so much more likely, and often results in us living life believing some very unhelpful things about ourselves. These beliefs result in a lot of negative emotion being triggered and mean we are much more vulnerable to emotional problems and difficulties with stress and anxiety.

To understand the second common problem, let's return to the idea of a self-esteem pie. Generally, as adults we get our self-esteem from a combination of these six factors, and life is fairly balanced. But for some people, self-esteem has come to be built with **too much dependence on one or two factors**. This is where personality can be a problem, as discussed in Chapter 9. If you happen to be very successful, the temptation is to build our self-esteem largely on that success (see the example in figure 11). But doing this makes us very vulnerable, and if that one thing is threatened, we will find that we experience a lot of anxiety and stress. A challenge to that part of our life has implications not just for whatever it was we were trying to do at the time but for the much bigger question of who we are. One person I worked with who had done this, building a self-concept almost entirely based on being good at everything she did, broke down when I asked who she would be if we took her out of a work scenario. 'I would be nothing,' she said, through her tears. This pressure can often result in a fear of failure and other issues such as workaholism or poor work-life balance, as we have to keep on that work treadmill in order to keep receiving this vital feedback that feeds our self-esteem.

Figure 11: Self-esteem based too strongly on one thing

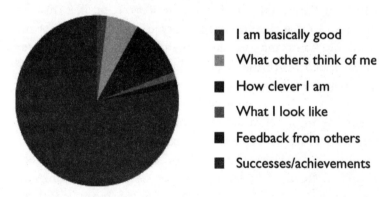

- I am basically good
- What others think of me
- How clever I am
- What I look like
- Feedback from others
- Successes/achievements

A third way in which self-esteem can be difficult comes from a similar issue, in which **one feature is over-influential**, but this time **affecting self-esteem in a negative way** rather than supporting the entire self-esteem. Here someone might have things they know are positive about themselves and would think that they were generally pretty decent if it weren't for one issue. That issue, often appearance, then dominates everything they think about themselves. So, because they are fat, ugly or thick, or whatever it is that they believe about themselves, their self-esteem is devastated and broken almost beyond repair, and nothing friends, family, loved ones or any degree of success anywhere else can do is able to change their view of who they are. It is as if their pie chart has become a Pac-Man, with that aspect of their self-esteem eating up anything else that might be positive (see figure 12). This can be very serious and, when it concerns feelings about appearance or weight, is often behind problems such as eating disorders.

Figure 12: Self-esteem eaten up by one thing

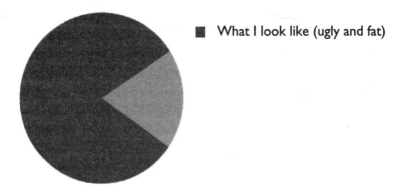

What I look like (ugly and fat)

Of course, the fourth thing that can affect our self-esteem in adult life is if we are unlucky enough to encounter **something that presents a dramatic and serious challenge to who we thought we were**. Often these are situations or circumstances in which something traumatic happens, and we are not able to control it or do anything to get ourselves out of it. These experiences challenge some of the most basic things we believe as adults: that we are in control of our own destiny and can protect ourselves and those we care about. They can bring home to us just how vulnerable we are. This alone is a serious challenge to anyone's self-esteem, but sometimes these incidents can bring an additional difficulty, especially if we feel that in some way an error or bad judgment on our part led to the situation. Anyone who has been responsible for a car accident knows the impact that has on them as they have to admit that they caused something very serious to happen. A severe challenge like that, even in adult life, can bring us almost back to square one, needing to build up our self-esteem from scratch. Just as difficult, though, can be a challenge from someone else. Being bullied is hard enough as a teenager, and it can be just as damaging as an adult; or a marriage that goes wrong, a boss who bullies and manipulates – these experiences can make us start to question the most basic things about ourselves, and this is a very stressful experience.

Difficulties with self-esteem, whatever their cause, are often very significant in problems with stress. Apart from being stressful in themselves, the extra emotions that are triggered, the unhelpful thinking patterns that often accompany low self-esteem and the impact that it often has on your life and relationships mean that stress easily rises to a level that is difficult to cope with.

So, how do you recognize low self-esteem in yourself? You may already be aware of it – perhaps your friends say that you do not value yourself as much as you should. Poor self-esteem can also show itself in our relationships, if we allow people to treat us badly and feel unable to defend ourselves, or if we feel that we do not deserve to be defended. Ask yourself: do you see yourself the same way as those who care about you see you? If they think you are wonderful and you do not, then the chances are that you could benefit from some work on your self-esteem, which may be making you particularly vulnerable to problems with stress and with difficult emotions. You might find it helpful to draw a pie chart like the ones in this chapter to think about where you get your self-esteem from. If you are building it all on one or two things, you are likely to feel very vulnerable, and if those things are ever threatened, you will most likely find that you experience some quite extreme emotions because those things are so important to you.

If you feel that a problem with self-esteem is part of the difficulties you are having with stress, be encouraged. Now that you know about it, you can start to do something about it! It is possible to rebuild self-esteem, even as an adult. Understanding how the experiences you have been through have led to your slightly wobbly self-image will help you to start to think about what the real truth about you might be. Do remember, though, that working through issues related to your self-esteem and self-concept is hard. It means taking apart the very foundation of who you are, so give it time. You need to be prepared to ask a lot of questions and look at the things you believe because it is likely that some of them are not actually true.

You can work through self-esteem issues with a counsellor or therapist. Ask your doctor if they can refer you or if they know any private counsellors in your area. There are also some good self-help books available that work on self-esteem issues using a CBT-style approach. One I would recommend is *Overcoming Low Self-Esteem* by Melanie Fennel.[1]

PART 3

Here and now

HOW TO DEAL WITH A HIGH-STRESS LIFE

12 What if you are at crisis point (or fear it might be just round the corner)?

So far in this book we've been focusing on understanding stress more – what it is, where it comes from and what might make some of us more vulnerable to it than others. I'm very aware, however, that, for many of you reading, stress is not just something theoretical or something that affects other people. Stress is an issue you are facing right now!

In fact, for most of us, stress is not something unusual or occasional. We do not just have the odd week or so when stress hits us, which we can navigate until the next calm comes. Many of us – and I include myself in this category – live a life where we negotiate with stress every single day. Every part of our lives – juggling work, family, friends, hobbies, pastimes, chores and responsibilities – involves decisions and actions that affect how much stress we are under. Twenty-first-century life is all about stress. On the whole, most of us would probably say that although stress bothers us, we are able to keep going in spite of it – we keep our heads just above water and push on until things calm down a little bit. But each and every one of us operating under this kind of stress risks a time when we start to find stress getting the better of us and having a very real and significant impact on what we are able to do. Ultimately, stress can have the power to stop us in our tracks.

Burn-out

Burn-out is a term used to describe what happens when we get exhausted – not just physically but also emotionally. It is a term used widely, although there are no specific diagnostic criteria. Burn-out occurs when our body and brain simply cannot continue functioning under the high demand and stress that has been the norm up to that point. Once again, it isn't about being weak and 'caving in'; it is a physical and psychological reality. You just cannot carry on under that level of pressure any more. If this has happened to you, don't feel bad or guilty that it happened. It is simply a sign that you are human, and recovery is not about 'pulling yourself together'; it is about getting some time away from that level of strain so that you can recharge and recuperate. It takes time.

Someone on the brink of burn-out feels worn out, physically and emotionally. They may have physical symptoms of long-term stress such as headaches, digestive problems or general poor health. Emotional symptoms are likely too, such as extreme mood swings with tearfulness or aggressive behaviour. Socially, burn-out leads people to struggle with things they would usually enjoy. Social occasions may feel like just one demand too many and the effort of keeping up a relaxed conversation just too much to bear. There are other symptoms. Often people at risk of burn-out are those in jobs that require them to give a great deal emotionally – very caring and supportive roles. These people are at particular risk both because their job inherently involves giving a lot out, which takes its toll over the years, but also because they are likely to be the kind of people who struggle with setting clear boundaries and getting clear time away from work. Quite simply, they care too much, and that leads them to keep working when they really need to be resting. If they are pushing the boundaries too hard, however, the very compassion that led them to that work in the first place starts to be eaten away. Bit by bit they start to care less, and eventually, as true exhaustion sets in, the bits of their job that used to stir them simply make them feel under more pressure. They no longer feel any sense of accomplishment or find a satisfaction in what they do. They have lost the spark of a job they used to love.

It's easy to talk lightly about burn-out, to joke about it with friends and colleagues, or to think that it is something that will never happen to us. But what if right now you are in the position in which stress has actually gone too far? We all have a breaking point – a point at which burn-out stops being something we live with and dice with week on week, and starts being something that has become a reality. No matter how much we would all like to think that we are immune to these kind of pressures and would never become ill ourselves, anyone can get to the point where the emotional, psychological and physical toll of stress means that we cannot go on – with work, or often with any kind of demand. It is as if the body finally calls a halt to things. People who have experienced full-on burn-out will talk of how they got to a stage where one day they just knew they couldn't do it – couldn't get out of bed, couldn't respond to their responsibilities, couldn't 'pull themselves together' any more. Of course, it isn't about pulling yourself together

– that's the problem. Burn-out is not something to do with being weak, lazy or overly emotional. It is a genuine physical condition in which long-term stress has taken its toll on us and we need time to recover – and it may take us by surprise. Listen to the experiences of Mark, a doctor, who found himself having to take time out from work to recover from burn-out:

'I never thought it would happen to me and I totally didn't see it coming. In my job everyone pushes themselves to the limit, and I wasn't unusual in working a lot of hours and not getting much time out. I've worked under a lot of stress for years so it wasn't anything new. I don't know really what pushed me over the edge that time. I'd been having some health problems – niggly things such as headaches, indigestion a lot and trouble sleeping. Things had been tough at home too – my long-term partner had got a new job that meant she was working away a lot and in the end we actually decided to split up, which was really hard. I was definitely feeling stressed – I found it really hard to turn off, was worrying about work even when I was at home, which I don't normally do. And when I was at work, my head used to race – it was as if the thoughts were going round so fast my head used to ache just with the pressure of all that thinking. I got to the stage where I was just going through the motions at work. I did the job but I didn't really care any more. In fact, I used to resent it if one of my patients didn't respond well to treatment. I took it personally and I hated that it meant I had to do more, or worry more out of hours. When it all came to a head, it was very sudden. I just woke up one Monday morning and knew I couldn't do it any more. I felt really stupid because I couldn't explain it, so in the end I called in sick and said I had a bug. But I went back to bed and just hid. I couldn't do it any more.'

Some of you reading Mark's story may well find that all of this rings true for what you are feeling right now. If things get to the extreme that Mark was describing, very often the only treatment at first is to take some time out, rest and re-gather yourself. It takes time for your body to recuperate and it is important you take that time. But often it is possible to do something before you get to that stage. Most people will find that they get some clear warning signs that stress is so high before they reach complete breakdown. The problem is that often we ignore those signs and carry on regardless. Some degree of burn-out isn't that unusual, and many people, particularly working in those very giving jobs, will find that they feel this way from time to time – often just before they take a long overdue holiday! It is easy to overlook those feelings and see them just as part of the job. Many of us expect that cycle of gradually getting more worn out and less motivated, then taking that long-needed holiday before returning to the job, trying to keep those feelings at bay. But burn-out is an issue we need to take very seriously.

Think about it this way. In certain professions, burn-out is one of the main causes for people leaving and moving on to something else. This means that for some people, the stress they currently manage day to day eventually drives them from a job they love and used to be committed to. Particularly if they work in one of those jobs in which burn-out is such a big issue, the way they handle stress might actually be one of the most significant things influencing how well they achieve in that career in the long term. This may be hard in the short term because they may have a genuine desire to do more, push themselves harder, go the extra mile. I have heard so many people say to me, 'Well, this is just what you have to do to do this job well.' But I say to them that working in a way that brings on symptoms of burn-out will only mean they do the job well in the short term. In the long term, they are likely to become more exhausted, more disillusioned, and eventually they may end up leaving.

So, if you really want to become great at what you do, take a good long look at how you can protect yourself from the stress it triggers.

This message is an important one for all of us, but it carries particular resonance for anyone who is working in a job in which giving of themselves – emotionally and physically – is a part of the job. Professions that involve this kind of giving – those with a high physical toll such as sporting careers, very physically demanding jobs or those that involve caring for other people or giving out to others and focusing on their needs rather than your own – are the professions for which burn-out is the biggest issue. Some studies of such professions found that half of the people who took part were at serious risk of imminent burn-out. Those most at risk are often those whose job is more than just something that brings in money; those whose job is a calling, a way of life, something that people love and is a huge part of who they are. These jobs include medical professions such as doctors and nurses and caring roles such as teachers, social workers and priests/ pastors. That is the tragedy of burn-out as it often affects the people who are most motivated by their job, most excited by what the job involves and most committed to what they want to do. These people, if they become victims of burn-out, have to deal not only with the physical and emotional effect it has on them, but also with the fact that they had to leave that job, that they will never achieve the things they longed to, and that the people they so wanted to care for now have to manage without them. They may keep trying to return to work but each time find the stress too much and end up taking further periods of time off. This repeated 'failure' – because that is what it feels like – can become added to the other worries and emotions that are part of the situation and end up having a very serious effect on that person.

What to do if you think you are at risk of burn-out

If you are on the edge of burn-out, or know that you are having symptoms of long-term stress in your life, it is important to take action fast. Be aware of the early warning signs of burn-out. Often the first thing people notice is that something of the love they had for the job has gone, some of their compassion has diminished. You may find that you are starting to think of the people you work with or care for as problems rather than real people, or that you simply don't respond to things that previously would have really got you excited or emotionally involved. You might start to worry about this and wonder why you don't care any more, but this can be the first sign that you have been trying to care too much. Other symptoms can include those in the list given in Chapter 6 – but it may well be that some of those symptoms have moved on from being occasional concerns and have become serious health issues. Mild headaches may have become regular migraines that stop you from working, or being a bit more prone to infections may have led to a serious long-term infection that you just don't seem to be able to shift.

If you have symptoms like these, then the first step is to get some help and check that there is nothing more serious going on physically – so do see your doctor. You may also be aware of things raised in part 2 that you think make you personally more vulnerable to stress. This next part of the book offers some practical ideas and takes you through some work you can do right now to help you to understand better why you are struggling so much with stress. It is worth discussing these with your doctor and looking into whether you can get some help or counselling. Most people who are referred to me because of problems related to stress do have something in who they are that is making them more prone to developing a problem with stress, and working through that certainly helps. Equally, however, I have never worked on stress management with anyone who has not benefited enormously from making some changes to their life and lifestyle that help them to deal with stress better. This part of the book is about the very important question of what you need to do in order to protect yourself from stress. This is not rocket science! Often there are simple changes that you can make which will help you right now to become more resilient to stress, and we'll be outlining some of these in the next few chapters.

Medication

A quick word on medication. Various medications are sometimes used for people struggling with symptoms of stress and/or conditions such as anxiety or depression. Very often people are resistant to taking medication. Some people feel that pills are not the answer, that they are an artificial 'solution'. Others are worried that they will end up having to take the pills for ever. Some people feel that there is a stigma associated with taking pills and don't want to take them for that reason. I can appreciate all of those worries, and I personally wouldn't want to take pills as though they were the only answer – they are not. But medication does have its place.

Think of it this way. Imagine life as rowing a boat across an ocean. Life is the ocean, and sometimes it is smooth, sometimes it is rough. On the rough days, waves sometimes come over the boat and you have to bail the water out. Some people, for whatever reason, also have holes in their boat. Maybe those holes are things that happened to them as children; maybe they are something life has thrown that damaged the boat. For whatever reason, their boat is damaged, so it lets water in and they have to bail out even more. If you are under a lot of stress, then you will have to do a lot of bailing over a long period of time, especially if there are holes in the boat letting in water too. Bailing in that way can get exhausting, and in a really rough time you might find that you cannot keep up. In that situation you might actually be at a very real risk of sinking under the weight of all that is going on.

What medication *doesn't* do is calm the water or mend any holes. Instead, it is a bit like having someone else alongside you for a while, bailing for you. This takes the pressure off and can reduce the risk that you will go under, bringing things to a much more manageable level. If it is just a storm that will blow over, medication can help you to cope while things are hard, and once they calm down you can gradually reduce the medication and stop. Medication can also give you a breather giving you the time and energy to do some work on mending any holes you have that might be making things worse. So, medication can be used alongside a therapy such as counselling or CBT, and it can make it much easier for you to have the emotional energy to look into what is going on beneath the surface in your brain. The medications prescribed now are not addictive and you shouldn't be on them for life. Medication should be about getting you through a rough spell or helping while you work on some other issues – so do ask your doctor if they can refer you for some counselling or CBT as well. Medication is particularly useful where certain symptoms are concerned, and specific anti-depressants have been found to be very helpful in calming obsessive anxious thoughts, for example, so if these are very much a feature of your difficulties, they may be suggested. Your doctor may also want you to consider taking medication if something that your stress is leading you to do might be dangerous – severe self-harm, for example, or if you are experiencing suicidal thoughts. Do be guided by your doctor but don't be afraid to ask questions and try not to rule out medication on principle. Used appropriately, it can make a big difference.

13 What to do – and what not to do!

Let's assume that so far reading this book you have become aware of the stress you are under – and perhaps of some possible reasons why it might affect you so badly. The next step, of course, is to look at some practical changes that can reduce the impact of that stress, or at least help to manage it so that it does not have such a great impact. This is particularly important if your job or lifestyle naturally brings with it a lot of stress, or if something about you or your personality mean that you are more vulnerable to stress or react more strongly to it. This chapter is about starting to make some changes and setting some things in place that will help you to cope with the stress you are under and minimize stress where you can.

First of all, it's worth saying something about some of the less helpful techniques people often use to try to cope with stress and why they do not work. You will remember from Chapter 7 that very often our natural tendency when we are experiencing a lot of negative emotion is to suppress that emotion and hope it goes away. Suppressing emotions is hard work and over time it does become more and more difficult. If you are someone who suppresses what they feel a lot, then you will be much more at risk of starting to use something else in an attempt to cope with what you are feeling. There are three main ways that people do this, and each of these can lead to causing more problems than it solves in the long run.

Alcohol and drugs

The first thing that people sometimes do is to turn to something that artificially counteracts their negative feelings, triggers some positive feelings and helps them to escape their stressful world for a while. Alcohol is often what is close at hand, but increasingly common is the use of recreational drugs such as cannabis, ecstasy, speed or cocaine. Using alcohol or drugs in this way often begins simply as part of socializing, and many people who have very stressful jobs will talk of the 'work hard, play hard' lifestyle. Of course, there's nothing wrong with having a social life, and if you do work very hard, then it is important that you have time to let off steam and chill out. However, be careful that what starts out as this doesn't become something you are using to try to cope with the stress of work. Although most of us would say that our own drinking is fine, around half of adults admit that they are concerned about the drinking habits of one or more of their friends.

Because alcohol is such an accepted part of our culture, genuine drinking problems can be missed. Alcohol is addictive, and using it to cope with stress can quickly become a problem. What starts as the occasional glass of wine at the end of a long day gradually turns into a few more each night, which becomes the bottle each night; that becomes occasional glasses at other times of the day when you are stressed, or something you need in order to get you through a stressful working lunch or difficult meeting. From that point, it is a slippery slope into alcoholism. The term 'alcoholic' often brings an image to mind of someone old, usually male, shabby, smelly and defiantly unwell. But there are huge numbers of what would be called 'functional alcoholics' in every town and city. These are people who habitually rely on drinking alcohol to help them cope and they consequently drink far more than is recommended each week. Drinking too much has serious health implications, and organizations involved with alcoholism are working hard to target these 'middle class' drinkers who are seriously risking their health. People who drink just twice the recommended limits (that is, 2–3 units per day for women and 3–4 units for men, with at least 2–3 alcohol-free days each week) are more than ten times as likely to suffer liver disease. It's not just the effect on your liver you should be aware of though, as drinking has been linked to other health risks, such as a striking increase in the risk of breast cancer (important information for the millions of women who drink more than the recommended levels each week).[1] Drinking too much also has a massive impact on relationships and the people you care about most.

Drinking too much and taking drugs obviously carry their own health risks, but the main thing in terms of using them to cope with stress is that it just doesn't work. Alcohol is a depressant, so in the long run people who drink to deal with stress feel worse rather than better. It interrupts their sleep, leaving them exhausted and chronically stressed. And the impact of those hangovers and worries about they did the night before can often trigger more emotion for them to have to deal with, which certainly doesn't improve their day. Most of all, even though they may have delayed having to face those feelings, they will still rise up eventually. Just like other ways of suppressing emotions, drinking or taking drugs simply doesn't work.

Another reason that people sometimes use alcohol or other drugs is to find artificial ways of relaxing and counteracting stress. Stress can push us to our limit and has been linked with more serious problems such as eating disorders and self-harm. All these things feel as if they might help in the short term but in the long term they certainly make things worse rather than better.

Scapegoats

Stress is something that causes a lot of negative emotions and generally makes us feel pretty lousy, but very often we feel powerless to do anything about it. A third thing that people turn to in order to try to feel better is attempting to change something else in the hope that it will make things better for them. It's as if that thing (usually something about themselves) becomes the scapegoat for everything else that is wrong (which they do not know how to change). Once you honestly believe that all your problems come down to that one thing, the solution feels simple – change that and all your problems will disappear. The most common scapegoat is something to do with weight or appearance. Many of us have got caught up in the illusion that if we can just control our weight and be slim – or even thin – then the rest of our life will also be better. Diet advertisements show people who have lost weight with miraculously transformed lives – they were once fat and miserable but now they are happy because they are thin! The truth is, of course, that losing weight (if we genuinely need to lose it) might improve some areas of our life but most probably the things that were making us really miserable will still be there. Millions of people in the UK alone have become caught up in cycles of behaviour concerning food and eating that leave them at risk of developing a serious eating disorder as they desperately try to solve the problems they have. Once again, trying to improve your life by blaming a scapegoat ends up causing many more problems than it ever solves.

'Work hard, play hard'

The final mistake often made in trying to deal with stress comes from the 'work hard, play hard' idea. As I have said, there are grains of truth in this and if you do work very hard, it is important to make time for yourself, time to let off steam and to relax. But many people – often those whose personalities make them prone to pushing themselves hard – fill their spare time with pursuits which, whilst fun, trigger almost as much adrenaline and stress hormones as the work they are leaving behind! An adrenaline rush can be addictive and the kind of sports that trigger it often also trigger endorphin release – the same hormones that are involved in making self-harm so addictive. Endorphins help us to feel more relaxed and positive and are behind the so-called 'runner's high', when people say they feel fantastic after a long hard run. These activities are great fun and certainly good things to do, but don't make the mistake of thinking that they are relaxing! Although they are a great distraction and relief for the brain from all the thoughts of work, and although the endorphins they release may help you to relax in the short term, in physical terms they still add to that baseline level of the hormones related to stress.

This kind of effect can be very subtle. Remember that stress is not just about being 'stressed out'. Even playing computer games – something many people do to get away from work and 'wind down' – actually requires a lot of concentration and attention, which to your body is a form of 'stress'. Or let's say you go away for the weekend – great fun but don't forget that the long drive (if that's how you get there) also involves a lot of stress from the perspective of both your brain and body.

So, what on earth *are* you supposed to do to handle stress positively?

The most important thing – more important than anything else – is to put into place times each week when you effectively and genuinely relax. We'll talk more about that in the next chapter as it's a topic in its own right, but a good place to start right now is to look at how you live your life and the boundaries you have between things that are stressful and things that are not. You need to take a kind of snapshot of your world. I encourage people to keep a diary for a couple of weeks of what they are doing each

Figure 13: Example of a diary

	Monday	Tuesday
12 a.m.	Sleeping.	Still awake, worrying about conference tomorrow. Get up and take herbal sleeping tablet.
1 a.m.		Still awake!
2 a.m.		Finally doze off sometime around this time.
3 a.m.		
4 a.m.		
5 a.m.		
6 a.m.		Alarm goes off. Oversleep as had bad night. Wake up at 7 when supposed to be leaving to drive to conference.
7 a.m.		Get dressed in hurry and drive to conference.
8 a.m.	Up, eating, getting ready for work, quick work call to check on details for presentation happening at 10.	
9 a.m.	At work, catching up on emails.	
10 a.m.	Morning meeting, give presentation.	Arrive (late) to conference. Miss half of first session and no time for coffee first.

hour of the day. Yours might look something like figure 13 below.

Once you have your diary for a week or couple of weeks, sit down with some colouring pencils or a highlighter or two. What you need to do now is to code each section according to whether it was work, leisure/'you' time, chores/getting something done that needed doing, or sleep. You might need other categories too – perhaps if you volunteer or do something in your evenings which isn't work but isn't leisure either, or if you have children or care for someone else in your family. Shade in your timetable according to those categories. This will give you a great illustration of where you give your time and energy at the moment.

11 a.m.		In conference.
12 p.m.		
1 p.m.	Working lunch, meet with colleague to discuss new project.	Conference lunch. Chat and network with other delegates.
2 p.m.		
3 p.m.	Catch up on some overdue work – try to get report done that was actually due on Friday. Try to get hold of someone on phone but with no luck.	In conference.
4 p.m.		
5 p.m.		
6 p.m.	Work phonecall – finally got hold of them.	
7 p.m.	Catch up on emails, note down main points agreed in phonecall.	Drive home.
8 p.m.	Go home. Takeout dinner and quick drink before throwing some clothes in wash as nothing to wear tomorrow and have important conference to go to.	
9 p.m.		
10 p.m.	Watch news, then check emails quickly before going to bed.	Totally worn out, have quick dinner then go to bed.
11 p.m.	Can't sleep, listen to radio for a bit.	Can't drop off, finding it hard to wind down. Listen to radio...

Once you have done this, try asking yourself the following questions:

The first is simple. **How much leisure/'you' time do you have in the average week? Do you ever 'stop'?** Very often we find that with the amount we have to do, this precious time can get pushed out. We cheat by filling it with other things, or with those things which although they are leisure, are actually physically stressful. A third of people admit that they hardly ever have any private 'me' time. Your body needs this space. Remember, it is about giving yourself a chance to lower those stress levels and return to that relaxed baseline. If you are one of the millions of people who never put in time specifically to relax, then make sure you read the next chapter carefully!

The second question relates to work. **How easy did you find it to define when you were and were not at work?** Some bits of the day are clearly work – usually that block of time in the centre of the day. In our 24/7 society, however, work has lost its clear boundaries. Unless you are lucky enough to have the kind of job in which you clock in and out and do no more work outside those hours, the chances are you will find your work creeping into what should be time for other things. Watch out for things such as the temptation to check your email out of hours. Yes, I know that your BlackBerry/iPhone/laptop/whatever it is (delete as applicable) is great because you can always be in contact with your work. But this means *you are always in contact with your work!* You never get away from it! This means you never properly switch off. This can keep your stress levels raised even when you are away from work. Remember that raised baseline stress and the effect that can have. It can contribute to problems with sleeping, interrupt family and leisure time, and increase your anxiety as you feel those emails hanging over you all the time. Around a half of adults admit they experience stress because they pick up emails out of work time or never turn off their work phone. You need to be able to get away from work in your 'down' time. If this is you, look at what simple steps you can take to try to put that boundary back in place. Do you really need to take your work laptop home with you at night? Must you keep your BlackBerry turned on in the evenings and at weekends? Can you look at getting separate mobile phones for work and for home calls so that you can make sure work does not intrude into your family or leisure time? Remember this is extra important if your job is stressful or involves a lot of giving out. If you do not make sure you have good regular time away from work, then in the long run you will risk burning out and not being able to do it any more. So, no sneaking a quick look at emails before you go to bed (is that really the best time to check work emails?), no taking non-urgent (and I mean 'life and death' urgent) calls in your evenings, no quick calls into work on your holidays 'to check everything is OK'. Give yourself clean boundaries and think: is this work time or not? The more you have messy boundaries and 'grey' part-work-and-part-free time, the more at risk you will be of stress.

The third question is about sleep. Sleep is a very valuable and elusive commodity for many of us, particularly those who juggle family with work and other demands. So, **roughly how many hours of sleep do you get each night?** Sleep is very important and very few of us get enough! Some interruptions to sleep are unavoidable (for example, young children) but do be aware that getting too little sleep will take its toll, so you need to try to counteract lack of sleep by putting in place some time somewhere in your day when you can relax and recuperate. Meanwhile, if you know that you are scrimping on sleep time because you are too busy, or if you are having trouble sleeping, do something about it! (See Chapter 17 for more on this.)

This is just the start of making some changes to your lifestyle and weekly timetable in order to make sure you are dealing with stress in the best way possible. Hopefully this exercise will have made you more aware of some areas you might need to work on. Suffering because of stress is not a sign of weakness. It is just a sign of being human. So, if it turns out that you, like me, are only human, try not to get caught up in an unhelpful coping strategy – something that will make things worse in the long term rather than better. Instead, put in place some space in which you can recover from the stress that life so often throws your way, deal with the boundaries and make sure that you keep some precious time for you.

14 Emotional gardening

So far we've been on a journey of starting to understand what stress is and how it affects us specifically. Hopefully, after keeping your lifestyle diary for a couple of weeks, you will have identified some areas in your life that may need attention. That, combined with the information you'll read in the next two chapters about introducing relaxation ('down') time into your schedule, will help you to start to make some serious changes to the impact stress has on you. But what about those of us who are experiencing more stress than it seems we should in the circumstances in which we're living? What if you feel you are not doing very much but are still struggling with experiencing a lot of stress? What if the chapters in part 2 have led you to suspect that there are some things about you and the way you approach life that may be making you much more vulnerable to stress than other people? Again and again research shows that individual factors such as personality and thinking styles can make all the difference in how much stress we experience. So, how do you start to look at the way you approach the world, and how do you change things about the way you think? This chapter will look at an exercise that will help you to start to become more aware of what is going on in your thoughts and emotional life when you are stressed.

Keeping a thought diary

This exercise involves keeping what is called a thought diary.

Thought diaries are all about looking consciously at thought patterns that would usually be automatic. Did you know that you are talking to yourself all the time? Some of us are more aware of our 'internal dialogue' than others, but we all do it! Thought diaries ask you to write down what your thoughts are at particular moments of the day.

When you are starting to investigate your own stress reactions, the best thing to do is fill out the diary each time you would say that you are feeling stressed. You can do this in the heat of the moment if that is possible, or fill it out at the end of each day, thinking back through the day to the times when you were stressed. Each time fill out the diary as follows (you can see an example in figure 14).

Start by noting the **time of day** you were feeling stressed and **what had just happened**. This is important because you might be looking for patterns in what triggers stress and because you want to know what you were reacting to. Next, write down **what emotions you are experiencing** and then **what you are feeling physically**. These two steps are important because sometimes we get so used to our emotional reactions that we don't even notice them. We notice feeling 'stressed' but don't pick up on the fact that it is because we are feeling anxious. Taking the time to ask yourself what emotions you are experiencing can help alert you to something like this, or you might notice that you are writing down the physical symptoms of an emotion like anxiety even though you are not aware of being anxious. The other reason this is important is because of the link between physical things and stress. You may note down something like 'having a lot of pain from my back' or 'have bad headache'. These kind of things over time might prove to have a regular pattern – perhaps because stress is triggering headaches you had blamed on something else, or because you are much more prone to reacting badly to something if a chronically painful condition is giving you problems.[1]

The next step in the thought diary is to **list the thoughts that are running through your mind**. Try to delve behind each one to see if something else is behind it that you are less aware of. You might write, 'I really mustn't be late for this appointment,' and miss the thought that lies behind it: 'What will they think of me if I am late? They might think I am incompetent!' Do practise this, and don't worry if you find it hard at first. Some people find it helps to think of their mind as a radio and to write down everything that is coming out of the speaker. Try not to censor what you are writing. It might be hard to put thoughts down on paper but you will get the best out of this if you are honest! You might also be surprised or even shocked to find yourself thinking some things. Don't judge the thoughts – just write them down! The interpretation stage follows on, but you won't be able to do it well if you haven't written down what you were really thinking!

Finally, note down in a final column **what you did as a result of what you were feeling**. This is very helpful as it might identify if you are reacting in ways that are unhelpful. You might even surprise yourself as you come to recognize what makes you do some of the things you do. Or you might realize that you do not do much in order to respond to your emotions. So where do they go? This might help you identify that you are at risk of not expressing your emotions, which makes you more likely to be suppressing them and which in the long term makes stress worse rather than better. This column can also be very helpful in the next stage when you are looking at introducing some more helpful responses into your life in those moments when stress takes hold.

Figure 14: Example of a thought diary

Where/ when and what has just happened?`	Emotions	Feelings	Thoughts	What did I do as a result?
3.30, Monday. Just dashed to a dentist appointment – was nearly 10 mins late as left work later than meant to and then also got stuck in traffic. Had to pay fine for being late and receptionist was very cross.	Upset at being told off. Stressed. Was really anxious when driving to appointment.	Hot and sweaty. Flushed. Bit shaky. (Embarrassed.)	I am so stupid. Why didn't I leave earlier? This is all my fault. This is just the start of a bad week – I bet it's all downhill from here. I bet that receptionist thinks I am a total waste of space. Or she thinks I just don't care and am lazy and slapdash. I should have been more assertive in talking to her. I am so useless at that kind of thing. I always make a mess of things.	Nothing really. I went back to work in a foul mood and was really ratty with a colleague. It did contribute to a very bad day though, so I opened a bottle of wine the minute I got home, which I don't usually do on a Monday!

The best thing to do is to fill out this diary each time you have an episode of feeling stressed over a period of a few weeks. From that you should have a set of diaries which you can then start to look at and take some time to analyse what you are thinking and feeling. Do remember, though, that it might take you some time to get used to filling out the diary, so don't rush yourself.

Once you have a reasonable number of examples in your diary, you can start to look more closely at the patterns in your thinking and in your experience. You might want to ask yourself the following questions:

Am I prone to any unhelpful thinking styles? Look through the lists of thoughts, and note down examples of unhelpful thinking as listed in Chapter 10. You might want to get a highlighter in a different colour for each one, and highlight any thoughts that are an example of that. There are a number of examples in figure 13. 'I am so stupid' is an example of emotional reasoning (you may feel stupid but that doesn't mean you definitely are), whereas 'This is just the start of a bad week – I bet it's all downhill from here' is an example of negative thinking (making negative predictions about the rest of the day and week based on one unfortunate event). The key with identifying these unhelpful patterns is to become more aware of when you are slipping into them. You will find over time that you notice yourself thinking in these ways in the moment, as it is happening. You might even be able to catch yourself and stop the thought before it comes out. It is important to realize that although it felt as if that thought was true, it probably isn't as bad as you thought.

Are there any rules or goals that I live by that are causing problems? Over time, as you keep an eye on your thoughts, you may find certain thoughts come up again and again. Often these will be examples of the unhelpful thinking styles, and it is almost as if they lie in the background, waiting for a chance to pop up and make you feel bad again! Some of these may have obvious roots in your past, but it may be more difficult to work out where others come from. One person I worked with found that time and time again the thought 'I am such a failure' came up in her thought diary. It happened in all kinds of scenarios, sometimes triggered by obvious things such as when she had messed something up, but sometimes occurring almost at random in circumstances when she would have expected to feel fine, such as when out with friends or when cleaning the house. If you identify a thought like that, it is very possible that this is linked to some kind of base belief you hold about yourself or about the world. Finding that belief is a bit like trying to reach down into the earth to find the root of a weed. This process is about looking through your thought 'garden' and trying to clear out any weeds.

I tend to use what I call the 'So what?' approach to do this. It goes something like this. You say (or write down) the thought to yourself. Then ask yourself, 'So what?' Try to answer quickly and instinctively – it's your gut reaction we want to access, not your more thought-through 'rationalized' thoughts. Keep asking 'So what?' until it feels as if you cannot go any further: you have got to the root. So, for the example above – 'I am such a failure' – you might go through a process like this:

'I am such a failure.'

SO WHAT?

'I always mess things up.'

SO WHAT?

'I'm always letting people down.'

SO WHAT?

'I should never let people down.'

SO WHAT?

'I should always be able to live up to what other people expect of me.'

SO WHAT?

'I should be a better person.'

Do you see how this process is starting to get from the thought 'I am such a failure' down to the rules that are at the root of it? In this case there are two beliefs that seem to be related to this thought – something about being able to be what other people expect and never let them down, and something about being 'a better person', someone who achieves very highly. The chances are that if you repeat this exercise with a few thoughts that seem to recur, you will find that some of them grow from the same root.

Of course, this exercise might bring out other things for you. You might notice certain patterns about when you feel stressed. Is it linked very much to certain people, for example? Or you might notice a link between your own stress and the way you respond. Perhaps you are more prone to being ratty or impatient when you are stressed. You might notice that you are not responding in a very positive way to stress (more about the right way to respond in the next chapter!). Hopefully, you will find this exercise a positive experience. It might be daunting seeing our thoughts and feelings down on paper, but understanding why we are feeling that way helps us to feel less out of control – and to see that it all makes sense! And if it all makes sense, there must be a way to change things that we want to change. I have never worked with anyone where, after this exercise and knowing their background, I couldn't say that what they were feeling was totally logical. It wasn't necessarily helpful or correct, but it *was* logical. Remember that this exercise is about understanding better what is going on. Avoid being tempted to place blame: this is not an opportunity for you to have a go at yourself or anyone else. It is simply an exercise in describing what is going on so that you can then decide what to do.

A word of caution

Before I move on, it's important to mention that for some people this exercise is very hard. They may be experiencing really intense emotions or struggling with very painful experiences or memories. Sometimes this process can lead them to dwell on those things or to feel trapped by memories and emotions that are retriggered by the process. If this is you, please don't persist in trying to work it out on your own. Identifying problem thoughts and the beliefs at their root isn't always easy, and many people find that it helps to have someone else's perspective on things. Think about sharing your diary with a trusted friend (perhaps you could keep diaries together and help each other to look at them), or go and get some expert help, either from your doctor or from a private counsellor. This isn't always something you can do on your own.

Whether you are working on your own or with someone else's support, once you have some idea of some of the thoughts that are troubling you, or the beliefs that are at their root, the next step is to start to challenge and question them. Understanding them has already stopped them simply being something automatic that you are unaware of. It gives you alternative options about how you might want to think or react. In fact, lots of us are living each day according to rules or beliefs that, if we thought about it, we don't even agree with! One quick test of this is to think about that rule/belief – for example, 'I should always be able to please everyone all the time.' Think of someone you love or care about and ask yourself, 'Would I teach that person to live according to this rule?' If the answer is 'no', then this raises the interesting question of whether you want to keep pushing yourself to live according to it.

Reforming unhelpful thought patterns

A longer version of this challenging exercise is to sit down with a piece of paper and think about why you believe that thought. Perhaps think of some examples of when you felt it, then try to write down what it was about that situation that made you think that thought. Think of it as writing down the evidence FOR that thought. You might put down things that people have said, or things that have happened, or things you have felt. Then think about whether there is any evidence AGAINST. Sometimes just outside of that particular emotionally charged moment we can see that actually things weren't so bad and the thought wasn't really accurate. Sometimes our friends and family actively disagree with the thought and we know they would challenge it. Try to think of any evidence against and then look at the overall picture you have – for and against. Your aim is to write down a more balanced conclusion. So you might write, 'When I realized I had burned the potatoes last night at the dinner party, I felt as if I was totally useless and never got anything right. Part of that came from feeling guilty because I felt responsible for the people I had invited having a good evening. But now I realize that a lot of why I felt that way was because of the pressure I put myself under to get everything perfect. In fact, people did have a good time in spite of what happened and, even if they hadn't, burning one thing doesn't mean I am useless. I cooked all the rest of the meal really well and everyone enjoyed the evening on the whole.'

This kind of 'reforming' of your beliefs is a very important step because these root beliefs often fuel the unhelpful thinking that can form the kindling for all those emotional bonfires. As well as stopping a belief from triggering so much emotion, you can stop it from forming kindling which can then burn into a bonfire. You might also become aware that some other things are linked to your own vulnerability to stress. So, as mentioned in Chapter 9, personality features are most risky if they become something you use in order to try to make up for a very rickety self-esteem – if you try to build your self-esteem on them. Someone who is a bit of a perfectionist will be all the more prone to starting to live life according to a rule that says 'I must always achieve highly at everything I do'. For that person, failing to do well at something not only triggers emotion because it contradicts the rule but also because it is the basis of their self-esteem. The threat of failure is a bit like someone taking an axe to the tree of their self-esteem and taking a great big chunk out of it – it's very risky. So, it makes sense that that person has developed a fear of failure, struggles to take criticism well, is prone to being over critical of themselves and so on. If we can deal with the root of the problem, which is the rule they live by but also the cause (their poor self-esteem), we will find that person suddenly has a lot less negative emotion in their life and, therefore, less emotional stress.

Of course, all of this takes time, so don't expect yourself to get it all figured out in a matter of days. In Chapter 10, I likened thinking styles to a dance that you have learned the steps to gradually throughout your life. You have been dancing it all that time, without realizing it. Changing those steps takes time. Changing the dance also can feel quite risky. The old dance wasn't great in terms of the outcome but you knew how the steps went and it felt safe and predictable. Once you start trying out new steps, you will find that that process in itself starts to trigger emotions such as anxiety because you don't know the outcome – you don't know how things will go or how people will react. At first, people might react badly as they are so used to you being the person they have known you to be. Give yourself time and be fair to yourself. This is not something to do in the middle of the most stressful period of your life! But if you can take some time to start to challenge things, you have the chance of releasing the potential within you as you escape from the limits that stress has placed upon you.

15 Learning how to relax

Now that we've looked at some simple dos and don'ts, and started to take some time to look at the thinking patterns that underlie our response to stress, it is time to move on and look at the big issue of relaxation. In many ways, this chapter is the most important of the whole book. It concerns something that is utterly essential for every human, something that we were designed to do but that many of us never do and often don't even know about. It is something that is utterly vital for children and teenagers to learn, but that very often the young people I work with have no idea how to do.

Relaxation is an essential part of the way that our stress system is designed to work. Remember in Chapter 3 how we looked at the natural ebb and flow pattern of stress, in which the spikes of stress then ebbed away, so that the baseline levels of stress remained low like water lapping at our feet? Relaxation is a way of spending time with no current stressors affecting us. It is a period of time when our sympathetic nervous system rests, and the parasympathetic can take the limelight and get on with the housekeeping jobs that it does, for a while not pushed into the background by the general stresses around us.

Relaxation is something that very often we need to learn, especially as life has become so much more vibrant, alive, 'in your face' and 24/7. Simple things can bring home to us how much more stimulating life has become even over the last few decades. Try watching an old video of a children's programme from 15 or 20 years ago. It is likely to be much quieter, much less vibrant and lively than children's television is now, quite often with longer periods of quiet when something is happening, but no one is talking and there is no music playing. These days, every space is filled with something to capture the child's attention. This means they are really well stimulated and learn a lot, but it also means that they risk losing their natural ability to relax and may need to learn or be taught just how important it is.

Effective relaxation

Relaxation needs to incorporate two things to be effective. Firstly, it needs to 'switch off' our brain and help us to stop thinking about the things that are stressing us out, put out any emotional fires smouldering and damp down any kindling-style thoughts that are lurking in the background. Secondly, it needs to help us to relax physically, bringing down the levels of stress hormones, relaxing muscles that have been tensed ready for action and lowering our heart rate and blood pressure.

Most people's immediate reaction when I start talking about relaxation is quite defensive. 'I'm not going to some relaxation class!' is often the next! Now, let me be clear: relaxation classes are fantastic and they are really good ways of relaxing. Many people love them (often, to be fair, these are people who would be good at relaxing anyway, or who have spent years learning how to relax successfully). However, for people who have perhaps never tried anything relaxing and live on a continuous adrenaline rush, they are like rushing from ten to zero in one go and will often prove impossible. In fact, trying hard to relax in this way can be really stressful! Don't worry: there are many more ways to relax than just going to a class!

Think about the things that people you know do to relax. We're going to make a list, so you might like to have a go yourself before you carry on reading. Think about friends, colleagues, people in your family. What kinds of things do they do to relax? Take some time to write your list, then read on – we're going to look at the most common categories of the things people do find relaxing:

The first thing people often think of is taking a bath! Taking a bath is a great way to relax for various reasons. First of all, it involves lying still somewhere that is nice and warm and generally quiet (as long as you can lock the rest of the family out!). This means that it involves **doing something that is naturally physically relaxing**. The warmth relaxes muscles, the calm helps to switch off anxious thoughts and the clear boundary means that you are leaving work behind (even that mobile phone or BlackBerry will have to be left behind so that it doesn't get damaged by the steam!). Of course, there are other things that fit in this category. Stretching out on the sofa next to the fire with a good book or going to the cinema to relax and watch a film are also examples of activities that are naturally physically relaxing, although neither is quite as good as a lovely hot bath!

We've already mentioned some examples of the next category. These are things that **absorb and distract your mind**. Things such as reading, watching TV or films, even cooking a complex recipe help you to relax because they switch your mind on to something else. This kind of escapism can be really positive and can help you to find pockets of time when you can have a respite from the thoughts linked with all the things you have to do. Some other examples would include things that take a lot of concentration and totally absorb your mind – perhaps practising a musical instrument or even knitting, sewing or doing embroidery. These can be very helpful, particularly if you struggle with anxiety or need to distract yourself from something that you are trying not to do. Distracting techniques are great because you can often combine them with something else – reading a book while in the bath, for example. Beware of the common pitfall though, because these often don't help to 'switch off' your mind. In fact, because they involve such a lot of concentration, some distractions are quite hard work! If you are trying to relax at the end of the day, trying to settle down before going to sleep, for example, you will need to make sure that you are not doing something that actually keeps you rather alert. Avoid the temptation to sneak work in around the edges, perhaps reading books related to work (management textbooks in the bath are not relaxing!) or books that take a lot of effort to understand and require you to use lots of brain power. The best things to read are those that don't need your brain much! There will never be a better excuse to buy trashy novels and magazines or to reread those books you love but know have little educational value! I have a library of Agatha Christies which I love to read when life is proving stressful – but each to his or her own. Find what works for you!

The third category is **sports or exercise**. Now, let's be clear here. Sports and exercise are very important and can be part of good stress management. Sport helps you to be less reactive to stress. Keeping fit and active reduces blood pressure, keeps your heart healthy and improves emotional well-being – it's a kind of stress antidote. It can also be a great way of getting rid of some of that physical tension. Remember how some emotions such as anger and frustration are very physical? Some sports are ideal if you have a whole day's worth of pent-up frustration because they give you the chance to 'act out' that aggression somewhere appropriate. A good hard run, a game of squash or a hard swimming session can all be great therapy! So it's good to make sure you exercise regularly. However, be aware that in the short term, a workout, a game of football or a day out mountain biking can actually create stress spikes as your body responds to the demands placed on it. Exercise is not the most effective form of physically relaxation in the short term, but it does form a vital part of your long-term stress management strategy.

Something often suggested, by women more than men, are strategies that involve **seeking social support**. Talking things through, sharing with someone else and hearing about their stresses and sharing yours are great ways of relaxing and de-stressing. We make the mistake of thinking that talking is only helpful if something changes or if someone produces a solution. The truth is that we were all designed to use talking as a way of helping us process difficult things that we have been through. Let me explain this with an example. When I was younger I used to do a lot of babysitting. One day a little boy I was looking after had a traumatic experience. He followed me into a walk-in cupboard and as I was trying to get something from a high shelf, a jar fell off and smashed on the floor next to him. For a toddler, this was pretty scary! He was very upset and took a long time to calm down. What was interesting, though, was what happened over the next few days. He took every opportunity he had to tell anyone he saw exactly what had happened (as best he could with very stilted language!). At first, telling the story seemed to upset him almost as much as it did when it happened, but bit by bit he seemed to be calmer when recounting it, and by the time he was telling a friend about it a couple of days later, he was even laughing and telling it as a funny story. This illustrates really well what our brain likes to do with something we have found hard. The process of talking about it gives us a chance to re-examine what happened. Other people's reactions also help us think about our own and how we might want to categorize the whole experience. Something about retelling and reliving what happened actually helps us to work out how to cope with it.

So, don't underestimate the power of sharing your day with someone else. Did you know you were designed with a basic need for the company of other people? A study of the behaviour of the chimpanzees at Chester Zoo in the UK found that after a fight other chimps would sometimes offer consolation to the victim. These caring gestures would usually come from chimps who were friends of the victim and would take the form of stroking, hugs or just some kind of play. This had an obvious effect on reducing signs of stress and distress in the other chimp. Being without this kind of good social support can magnify the impact of stress. People who are handling a lot of things on their own are most at risk – single parents or those who are not married or living with anyone, for example. Particularly if you feel quite isolated, take some time out to look at your friendships. How many people do you have around you whom you can call on for support when you need it? Some people are really good at being a support to others but are not so good at asking for help themselves. Don't neglect this method of dealing with stress. Get together with friends for coffee or, if you cannot get out, call someone or join an internet forum. And remember, if someone is talking things over with you, you don't have to feel under pressure to come up with some amazing solution or suggestion. The basis of counselling revolves around supporting and giving people space to talk about what they have been through without offering solutions or suggestions. It really is good just to share!

In a way, what this sharing offers us is some support in doing the next thing that can be a great way of de-stressing. This is all about **getting difficult thoughts, experiences and emotions out of our heads and changing our thinking**. Remember that some unhelpful patterns of thinking actually make emotions – and stress – worse. So often our reaction to something that happens can trigger stress when in reality things are not as bad as they seem. Ultimately, what CBT does is help us to learn to get rid of unhelpful thinking and replace it with things that help us respond more positively to stressful situations. Think about it: there are actually two ways to respond to anxiety. Let's say you are about to get married. Most people find they are pretty nervous, but it's a positive thing and that nervousness is tangled up with excitement. So, you respond to the anxiety by gritting your teeth, smiling and going on with what you were planning. This is very different to the kind of anxiety that is crippling, that makes you want to run and hide. The key, of course, is to do with how in control you feel, but your attitude to anxiety is also important. Very often it is the fear of fear that does a lot more damage than fear itself!

Friends can be very useful here too, helping us to think more positively, challenging our less rational fears and helping us to think things through. Also useful, of course, is more formal help such as CBT. But don't forget little things you can do to get rid of unhelpful or incessant thinking.

Little things can be very helpful, particularly if you have a lot of thoughts buzzing round your head. Something as simple as writing them down can help. Think about it: how many times have you gone to the supermarket with five or six things in your head that you must remember? As your brain detects how important they are, it sets them on a constantly circulating loop in your mind. This takes a lot of energy and is stressful (and you usually end up forgetting one anyway!), so why not just write them down? If you are lying awake thinking of things you need to do the next day, write them down. Then you will not have to remember them and your brain will not keep being lurched out of sleep as another thought pops to the surface. Sleep therapists often suggest keeping a notepad by your bed so that you can jot down thoughts that occur to you and do not have to try to hold them in your mind.

The final thing that can help us relax is **using things that aid relaxation.** This is all about making your surroundings more relaxing so that it is easier for you to relax. If you are trying to have a half-hour of relaxing, you'll find it pretty difficult if there are people walking through the room you are in, if it is very bright or noisy, if there are distractions around such as phones ringing. Certain things can make an environment more relaxing – some kinds of music, appropriate lighting, or using candles, for example; things such as aromatherapy oils genuinely help you to be more relaxed. These methods are things to use in conjunction with something else. So, why not light a candle or put some chill-out music on while you take that bath? It's about making it as easy as possible to relax. You could even book yourself in for a regular massage or even acupuncture, both of which aid relaxation.

So, these are the main categories of activities and things that can help people to relax. How many ideas did you get? Can you now think of any more things you might be able to try? These things are also great strategies for lifting your mood if you are feeling low or dealing with something such as anxiety. Remember, though, that it is about *learning* to relax, so the first time you try something you may not find it very relaxing. Take your time and try lots of different things from your list several times. You might find it helpful to note down what works and what doesn't work and why. Be creative – try different things and start to work out what is right for you. Everyone is different.

Learning to relax is about gradually finding out how to switch your body and mind off and bring that stress baseline back down to normal. Once you get better at it, you will find that it is much easier and you will not need to be as deliberate about it. But for now, you will need to schedule in specific periods of time for 'relaxation practice'. Remember, this is important! Although it might feel as if you are doing nothing, planning relaxation is the most important thing you can do to make sure that you are able to keep doing everything!

16 Fitting relaxation into your life

After the last chapter you should have a good list of things you could do to practise relaxing. Now though, let's look at the practical question of when on earth you are going to do them! This chapter is about how to fit relaxation into your life because that is what this book is all about: not just understanding more about how stress affects you but taking some time to think about what you are going to change as a result.

If you do only one thing as a result of reading this book, work out how to fit in some regular relaxation. There are many myths about relaxation, and because of some of the classes and techniques around, some people see it is a rather 'New Agey', 'alternative' thing to do. You know the kind of reaction – 'It's nice, and some people like it, but it's not for me.' But relaxation is actually essential for all of us, whoever we are, wherever we come from and whatever we do. Some people are naturally really good at relaxing. Their personality is more laid back, they tend to be less prone to anxieties and they suffer less with stress. But if you are not one of those people, this isn't an excuse for you to rule relaxation out. It simply means you have to make more of a deliberate effort to relax regularly.

How often?

People often ask how often they should be relaxing. The

truth is that every day should include a slot of time for you to chill out a little. You might put this at the end of your day or you might take an hour or so out after you have just done something particularly stressful – maybe a difficult presentation, class or meeting. Try to make it a regular slot, something you do each day after work. Think of relaxation as the antidote to stress.

Let's be realistic. You may have one of those weeks from time to time (or more often!) when you barely get a chance to stop at all. Or do you have days like I do when you can get right through to six or seven in the evening before you have time even to stop for a cup of tea or something to eat? If you know you have had a hard day or week, then remember that means you need to relax. You can think of it as a bank account. If you imagine your energy reserves are the amount of money in the account, a busy day or week is a bit like constantly taking money out. Relaxing is when you put money back in. So, if you have had a really busy time, making lots of withdrawals, you need to spend some extra time relaxing and balancing that out. If you know in advance that you are going to be busy, you can even plan something relaxing at the end of that busy period.

At first when you start making time to relax, you may find it hard to think of what to do, or find that you feel guilty for stopping and 'doing nothing'. Remember, though, this is not time doing nothing. It is time relaxing, and thereby enables you to do all the other things you do in the day. Without it, you will end up doing much less in the long term. The trick is to treat learning to relax in much the same way as you would learning any new skill. Come at it from a position of being fairly analytical. Try lots of new things and note the effect they have on you. Most of all, give it time.

You will not learn to relax overnight, and at first you may find your mind jumping back to work, or you may feel the urge to get up and do 'something productive' or deal with something you know needs doing. But relaxation is really important, so remind yourself of that and stick to what you have planned.

Planning relaxation

So, let's start to look at how you are going to introduce more relaxation into your day. First of all, get out the timetable you kept as part of Chapter 13. You need to work out how you are going to fit some times for relaxation into your day. This might mean making some changes. You might need to leave work slightly earlier, get a dishwasher or move some commitments around. You might even find at first that you need to shed some of the things you do. This might seem counterproductive. But remember that, ultimately, learning to relax is something you need to do in order to be able to keep pushing yourself hard and fitting so much into your life. Although there may be a period when you have to slim down what you do for a while, you should find that eventually you can take those things back on. Do remember, though, that you are only human! Sometimes it may be simply about admitting that, much as you would like to, you cannot do everything.

When planning how much time to relax, don't aim too high at first. As you get more used to including relaxation in your everyday life, you'll find that it is automatically built in. Right now you may find that three or four half-hour or 45-minute sessions each week is all you can fit in. If you can, try to get something in every day. You may find that on some days you have no time, whereas on other days you can take a whole morning or afternoon. That is fine. Eventually you will be doing things to relax much more automatically and you won't have to do this 'scheduling'. At first, however, it is important; otherwise you'll find that it just gets pushed out and you'll have gone through the whole week and not done it. So, think about your next couple of weeks and plan when you will fit in your relaxing time. I would suggest you actually write it down because this makes it more likely that you will stick to it.

The best way to start is to put together a list of ideas of things you could do to relax, just as we have done in Chapter 15. Use the categories in that chapter to help you if you haven't already written your list, but also think about what people you know do, or things you would like to have time to do but never manage to fit in. Get as many ideas as you can and try to be varied. Include some things that you can do at home and some that involve going out; some that involve other people and some that are just you on your own; some that are shorter and some that take up an evening or few hours. Have a brainstorm and write down as many ideas as you can (you should have at least ten). So you might put 'have bath and read book; watch episode of *Friends*; meet friends for coffee; go and watch film at cinema; go for long walk; play round of golf...' and so on.

Write down your ideas in the box opposite. (If you are really good at this, you might need more space, so do use another piece of paper!)

Space for your list

Once you have your list, you are ready to go. For each 'relaxation slot' in your week you need to select one thing from your list. Obviously it needs to fit the slot you have available, but do try each thing on your list at least once. Once you have started, make sure you do it for the allotted time, even if you don't feel like it! Make a note in the table below of what worked and what didn't, and why. You might want to give each activity a score out of ten for how successful it was in terms of relaxing. This way, you can gradually learn what works for you and get better and better at it. So you might write, 'Monday 8 p.m. Bath for half an hour with book. 7/10.

Enjoyed book, but kept getting interrupted by children with their homework. Next time do later once children in bed.' Or, 'Friday 1–2. Played tennis over lunch with colleague. 3/10. Nice to have the exercise but was very wound up by work so kept hitting balls out. Got very frustrated. Next time maybe play squash as it is a bit more forgiving.'

Record of relaxation experiments

When?	What did you do?	Marks out of ten	Notes/comments

Once you have tried all the things on your list, you can start to fine-tune it. Gradually aim to get a good idea of what works for you – then practise it! Remember, relaxation is a skill you will learn, so it does take time. Even the perfect relaxing activity for you might not work brilliantly at first. You have to give it time! These tools are your main weapon against stress, so be determined!

Relaxation exercises

A final word on relaxation exercises before we finish. They can be tricky and take some learning but they are excellent ways to relax physically. They can be particularly helpful if you struggle with anxiety or specific problems such as insomnia or panic attacks. So do not rule them out. Perhaps include them as part of your list and give them a go once you have started to get better at relaxing. Or set yourself the task of doing a relaxation exercise, but make sure you persist with it! Don't forget that at first you will find it hard; it is a skill just like anything else. You might be able to learn a technique, so look into local lessons. Whatever you do, practise, and remember that the more you do practise, the more effective it is likely to be.

It is worth learning a short and simple relaxation exercise. This is one I recommend and it is something you can do wherever you are, whatever is going on. It is short, simple and quick and will help you to regain your cool if things are stressing you out. It can also help to settle anxiety or hold off symptoms of panic and help you to stop your head from exploding on those days when things just seem to keep coming at you non-stop.

At first, like all things relaxing, this will take some practice, so bear with me. You need to find a song or piece of music that you like and find relaxing. If it has words, choose one with words that are comforting, soothing or calming. You might want to choose something that reminds you of a time or place where you felt safe or calm or of people who care about you and give you lots of support. Find a quiet place where you won't be disturbed. You need to put that song/piece of music on repeat on your CD player or mp3 player. Put it on, sit (or lie if you prefer) comfortably and either close your eyes or let yourself stare into space (some people don't like to close their eyes but it does help to block distractions). Listen to the song and either sing along quietly or hum the words. This may feel odd to you, but it is important as it helps you to regulate your breathing and stops you from over-breathing, which is something that makes the symptoms of anxiety and panic worse. Sing or hum your way through the song two or three times. As you do this, imagine that every time you breathe in you take in clean, calm air. As you hum and breathe out, the stress is blown away, to be replaced by that clean air. Try to focus on the song or tune and forget what is around you.

Repeat the exercise as often as you can – at first a few times each day – with the same song. The more you practise this when you are feeling relatively calm, the more effective it will be. The key is that you will begin to associate that song with being relaxed. Eventually, once you have practised it enough, just hearing the song will help you to start de-stressing. The breathing exercise will also help to calm you down. If you are out and about, or at work or wherever, and start to feel stress rising and threatening to overwhelm you, you can find somewhere where you can have a few minutes of peace (even popping to the loo can work!). Sit and close your eyes and hear the song or tune in your head. If you are somewhere private, you can hum along; if not, then breathe as though you were humming with nice long breaths out. If you have an iPod or mp3 player, you can even keep the song with you and actually play it to yourself. Repeat the song a couple of times until you feel able to go back into your day.

Of course, you can do this with more than one song (the first might start to drive you mad after a while), but keep it to two or three. Remember, you need to associate the songs with those times when you are somewhere safe and secure, and totally relaxed and chilled out.

17 Dealing with sleep problems

Before we finish, I must mention problems with sleep. Of all the problems most commonly associated with stress, sleep is the one that most of the people I support struggle with. In fact, most people I know admit that they are usually tired. The most common response I get to the query 'How are you?' is 'Tired'! Many people, living in a 24/7 society and often frantically juggling many different responsibilities as well as trying to fit in a social life, find that sleep is the thing that gets squeezed out. The problem is that sleep is very important – more so than we might think – to both our physical and emotional well-being. In recent years, as we have come to understand more about sleep, there have been many studies looking at the effect of lack of sleep on our physical and mental health. Most studies seem to find that that the ideal amount of sleep health-wise is between seven and eight hours each night but that only one in five of us manage to achieve this. It isn't just the adults struggling, either. A third of teenagers (often maligned for sleeping too much!) admitted that they only slept for an average of between four and seven hours per night, and, of course, sleep problems in younger children are one of the most common behavioural issues that parents seek help for.

What if you don't manage to get that level of sleep each night?

Apart from being a bit drowsy, what might it do to you? Just like stress, the impact lack of sleep can have is quite surprising – alarmingly so if you are one of the millions of people who tend to burn the candle at both ends. If we sleep less than recommended, there are studies suggesting we might be more susceptible to a whole variety of health problems, including colds and other infections, hardening of the arteries, heart problems, even Type 2 diabetes. In fact, if we get very little sleep – around five hours or fewer a night on average – we might even be risking our life. Studies suggest that the risk of death from heart problems is doubled if we exist on this little sleep in the long term.

Meanwhile, of course, not sleeping affects the way we react to things and the way our brain works the next day. So, if we are sleep deprived for whatever reason, although we will find we have some periods of time when we operate reasonably well (almost as well as if we had slept properly), the chances are that in between those moments of clear thinking we are likely to struggle with issues such as poor concentration, slow responding (that classic effect where we feel as if we are operating on a time lag!) and, of course, drowsiness. This is a serious risk if your job is potentially dangerous or requires good concentration for long periods of time – for example, if you do a lot of driving or operate machinery as part of your job, or if you are caring for other people. There have been well-documented reports of exhausted doctors and nurses making potentially fatal errors with drug prescriptions, measuring doses or just not picking up on important signs and symptoms. Sleep deprivation has been blamed for several major incidents, from car and rail accidents to major disasters such as the nuclear meltdown at Chernobyl. If sleep deprivation carries on for too long, it can lead to hallucinations and serious problems. People who have tried to stay awake for as long as possible find it harder than you might think, and *Guinness World Records* has actually taken the 'staying awake' class out because of health risks. (If you are interested, the record before they removed the class stood at just over eleven days and nights without any sleep!)

Of course, it's not just about how well you will work if you are not sleeping. Poor sleep also seems to affect the way we see the world and react to it, affecting the way we interact with other people, react to circumstances and challenges during the day, and how we feel in ourselves. Lack of sleep has been shown to make people more likely to respond in very emotional ways to certain situations or images, with emotions such as anger and sadness in particular much more likely if they are very tired. Most of us have been there and recognize how much less well we deal with things and control our emotions and reactions, and how much more prone we are to blowing things up in our own minds (slipping in to some of those common thinking errors discussed in Chapter 10) and overreacting. So our lack of sleep can very often affect other people as well as ourselves!

Why exactly is sleep so important?

It has been something of an enigma to scientists for a long time, but recently our understanding of its role has been developing. In fact, various significant roles, purposes and processes are now proposed and debated by professionals from different specialities and backgrounds. Sleep certainly does much more than just rest our bodies physically. Although we may not understand exactly what its purpose is, what we do understand is that it is very important and plays a role in keeping our bodies and minds healthy. Sleep seems to be important for rest and repair, and for other important processes that need some time when they can happen 'in the background'. Although some parts of the brain switch off almost completely while we are asleep, others remain remarkably active, and sleep seems to have a role in strengthening connections between some nerve cells in these regions. This evidence has backed up those theories that have long since suggested that sleep helps with processes such as the consolidation of memories or things we have learned. A good night's sleep really does affect the way our brain works the next day, and people who have had a good night's sleep perform better on tests of memory and reasoning or logic skills. This is particularly important, therefore, at times when you are learning a lot, and, predictably, lack of sleep seems to adversely affect academic performance.

So, if you are sleep deprived, what is the most likely thing to be causing your problem? First of all, of course, there are some things that simply don't let you sleep. Anyone with small children (or sometimes even older children!) might find that this is significantly limiting the number of hours they might be able to sleep; at the times they feel able to sleep (at night), their children don't seem to find themselves in the same position and therefore keep them awake. Other things can keep us awake, of course. Anyone who has a partner who snores will be able to sympathize with this plight. In fact, three-quarters of British adults snore and one in three snores so badly that it keeps their partner awake.[1]

Aside from these things, if there is one thing that affects our sleep, it is stress. Having a difficult time at work or in another area of our life is often something that can leave us lying awake many hours after we have gone to bed, struggling to turn our mind off. Anxiety is a particular bad guy where sleep is concerned. It's probably not surprising that Sunday is the most common night for people to say they have slept badly, and Friday night, with the weekend offering a rest from work thoughts, is the most common time for people to have a good night's sleep. Research suggests that as many as 23 million people working in Britain lose sleep because they are worried about work the next day. Issues such as dealing with a difficult boss or challenging colleagues, having to give a presentation or lead a meeting the next day, or missing a deadline are all common causes of lost sleep.

It is unfortunate that stress is so prone to affecting our sleep because in fact sleep is a very important part of our arsenal against stress. If we tend to push ourselves and work under quite stressful conditions, sleep is one of the golden opportunities we have to recuperate and try to avoid that stress having a long-term impact. It seems that sleep has a role in counteracting the stresses of our day. So, for example, our blood pressure naturally falls when we are asleep, as do the levels of some of the stress hormones. Sleep seems to offer a natural chance to rest, unwind and bring that stress baseline down ready for the next day. Sleep also helps to counteract some of the metabolic impact of stress. This means that if we do not get enough sleep, we are at a greater risk of weight gain and even of obesity as a result of stress. This isn't anything to do with how many calories we use up (because, in fact, we use fewer when sleeping); it is because sleep is one of the natural systems that rebalances some of the changes stress brings into our system. Even young children seem to be affected by this, with those who are poor sleepers more likely to have problems with gaining weight and risking childhood obesity. Lack of sleep causes a rise in the hormones and processes triggering stress... which means that it is harder to sleep... which can mean another rise in stress – it's easy to see how the vicious cycle of insomnia develops.

So, sleep is very important and we should all make time to have our recommended seven or eight hours a night. Of course, it is not as simple as just making sure we are in bed for that length of time! Quality of sleep is also important and it is only those who say that they spend over 90 per cent of the time they are in bed actually asleep who seem to reap the health benefits. Some of the studies looking at the health impact of lack of sleep have found that even if you did have *enough* sleep, if you lacked a certain kind of sleep – the deep sleep that seems to give time for those restorative processes to occur – the health risks persisted. We need to learn to sleep in order to protect our health from the impact of stress – but we also need to learn how to sleep *well*.

Sleep problems are one of the most frustrating things to suffer with. We all know how easy it is to start to find sleep difficult, because it is such a psychological thing as well as a physical phenomenon. Very often, as soon as we start to find ourselves thinking, 'I bet I won't get to sleep for ages tonight,' it comes true. This is why, on the whole, doctors advise against using sleeping tablets too often: it is very easy to come to depend on them, physically or psychologically, and then to find sleeping without them really difficult, particularly when, as happens with most sleeping tablets, they start to become less effective as time goes on.

Improving your sleep

So if you are one of the 10–15 per cent of the adult population suffering with long-term or chronic insomnia, what can you do to try to improve your sleep? The most important thing is to try to harness the natural systems in your body that control your sleep–wake cycle. Your brain controls this natural rhythm with a group of cells that automatically 'tick' and seem to operate roughly on a 24- or 25-hour cycle. This, along with changes in certain hormone levels, controls when you would normally wake up naturally or feel sleepy. Your body works to a natural, predictable rhythm: you start to feel sleepy, so go to bed and to sleep at roughly the same time each evening, then, due to hormones released at the right time, you naturally start to become more wakeful at a certain time, hopefully when you want to get up! This is why if you usually get up at seven for work in the week, you might find yourself irritatingly alert by half past seven or eight o'clock in the morning even on those weekends when you plan to lie in. Your body is primed to get up at that time![2]

This means that we benefit from having a sleep cycle that is as regular as possible. Your body does naturally sleep reasonably well, so if you are finding it hard, work with it and use its natural systems to help you sleep. Try to go to bed and to get up at the same time each day. This is particularly important if you are not sleeping well. Many people get into a pattern of going to bed at a certain time, but find they cannot drop off until the small hours and so often sleep late in the morning to catch up on lost hours. What this means is that initially frustration is keeping you awake, but gradually your sleep–wake cycle shifts so that your natural sleeping time is, say, from 4 a.m. to 10 a.m. Although this might feel as if you have had a dreadful night – and it would certainly be pretty frustrating if you went to bed at 11 p.m. and spent five hours awake – you actually slept for a reasonably good six hours. Solving this kind of sleep problem is often about making yourself get up in the morning so that you avoid shifting your cycle later and getting your sleep at the wrong end of the night. Experts advise that you look at how long you successfully sleep (in this case those six hours), then go to bed at an appropriate time that allows you just those six hours (plus a bit of time to drop off) in bed. At first, for example, you might go to bed at midnight and set the alarm for six. If you make yourself get up – even though you will still struggle to get to sleep and may actually get very little sleep for the first few nights – gradually you will find that your natural sleep pattern moves back to a more helpful time. Once that has happened, you may well find that you can extend the time and allow yourself to sleep in a bit more, meaning you spend more time asleep.

Of course, the biggest problem affecting sleep is often those incessant thoughts that just keep buzzing round your head. If you struggle with stress, or anxiety in particular, this is likely to be something that contributes towards your problems with sleeping, and once you have started to find sleep elusive, thoughts and worries about whether you will manage to sleep are added to those and make things worse. Cognitive Behavioural Therapy, already mentioned in relation to unhelpful thinking patterns in Chapter 10, has been shown to be very effective in dealing with this kind of problem. In fact, one clinic claims that if CBT is done well, about 80 per cent of people suffering with insomnia will see an improvement after just five sessions. Don't be afraid to go to your doctor and ask for a referral to a psychologist or CBT practitioner for help with your sleep problems. The sooner you start to tackle the problem, the sooner you will find yourself more able to get back to sleep!

More practical tips to help you sleep

- Think about how and when you are going to fit sleep time in and give yourself some time to prepare for sleep. Don't expect to go straight to bed from that lively work meeting that finished late. Give yourself an hour or so to wind down, perhaps reading, taking a bath or doing something else you find relaxing. This will help you drop off when you do eventually go to bed.

- Avoid alcohol and caffeine if you want a good night's sleep! Although alcohol might help you to drop off, it stops you from having those all-important deep sleeps, meaning that you wake more and end up feeling much less refreshed the next day. Caffeine makes it much more difficult to drop off and can stay in your bloodstream for a surprisingly long time. If you struggle with sleep, avoid caffeine for several hours before bedtime. People who are very sensitive might find that they need to cut it out all together for the sake of their sleep.

- Banish mobile phones from your room or at least switch them off! Apart from the chance that someone will text you in the middle of the night and wake you up, research suggests that something from the radiation released by mobiles can affect your sleep, disrupting deep sleep or simply keeping you awake.

- Tempting as it is, try to avoid going to sleep with the TV or radio on. Although you will be sleeping, you will not go into the proper deep sleep you need. This results in what some experts call 'junk sleep', when you are sleeping but not in the way that is good for you!

- Avoid napping in the day if you possibly can. If you must nap, keep it short and try to grab what are called 'power naps' – 20-minute quick naps or periods of 'shut eye' that some claim can be as effective as sleeping for several hours!

- Try to keep your bedroom quiet, not too hot or cold, and nice and dark. One thing that changes as we get older is that we tend to sleep more lightly, meaning we are more easily disturbed by noise or light. This can lead to more waking in the night, which, if you are feeling under stress, can then give you the chance to get your brain going again, making it very difficult to fall back to sleep!

- If you cannot sleep, don't lie in bed for ages waiting to drop off. No, it's true: no matter how counterproductive this might seem, all research shows that if you do this, you are likely to get frustrated and this will in itself hold off sleep. It is tempting to think that if you stay there, you might just drop off, but most experts suggest you give it perhaps 15 minutes to half an hour. If you still don't feel sleepy, get up, go somewhere quiet and do something restful such as reading until you feel drowsy, then return to bed when you feel as though you might drop off.

- If there are any other problems affecting your sleep, such as recurrent nightmares, serious snoring (sometimes called sleep apnoea), other physical health problems or practical things such as having to get up to pee a lot in the night, do go to your doctor and discuss them. There might be something else affecting your sleep that can be treated.

Conclusion

I've lost count of the number of people who, on hearing I was writing this book, have asked me if I am finding it stressful! But seriously, I find myself finishing this book at a time that for me, as usual, has been one when stress has presented a pretty significant challenge! I guess many of us will never eradicate stress completely from our lives. In the same way that we will never be able to rid ourselves totally of those internal gremlins that make us prone to unhelpful thoughts, difficult emotions or stressful moments, stress will inevitably always be there to some degree.

Ultimately, I think that is the most important thing to learn about stress. We should never allow ourselves to become complacent and ignore stress, pretend, it isn't there or won't affect us, and hope it goes away. Remember, learning to deal with stress is about a lifelong journey of becoming better at handling it, but also learning to spot stress more quickly before it starts to become a problem. Successful stress management, like managing our weight, isn't about short-term regimes that are impossible to maintain. It's not about short periods when we manage to relax enough, live reasonably healthily and hold it all together until the next time things go crazy and it all goes to pot. Stress management is like learning to 'eat healthily' all the time. It is about fitting relaxation and 'down time' into our daily and weekly schedules so that stress is never allowed to get a foothold.

We should be aware, however, that we probably won't get it right all the time. Healthy eating includes periods of time when we indulge ourselves, and dealing with stress is the same. We will all have times where just by chance life throws a whole bunch of stuff at us that places demands on us (why do those things always seem to all happen at the same time?). In those moments, the better our skills of stress management and the greater our arsenal of anti-stress weaponry and relaxation methods, the better our chances of getting through it without going crazy at some point (or driving those around us crazy instead). I have learned never to scoff at or rule out anything that is recommended to me as being useful for dealing with stress. It is always worth looking into things and, if we are happy with what is proposed, giving them a try! The worst that can happen is that they don't work. Life needs to be a journey of adding to the things that we know help us when things have become stressful – when suddenly the water levels are around our neck and we are starting to feel that sense of fear that we might go under.

I hope that this book has been a helpful step on your journey. Do keep learning about stress and adding to what you find works for you in terms of coping with it better. If you have identified that there may be things making you more vulnerable, keep looking into them. You deserve to reach the potential that you have, and stress, of all things, should not be allowed to stop you! Use the other people you have fighting on your side. Talk to your doctor, share ideas with friends – even consider joining a relaxation class. You won't manage to get things perfectly right as a result of reading this book. Neither will I! I guess we'll all have days where stress gets on top of us, but, hopefully, we will be able to learn a way of managing life in the challenging world we live in without stress seriously affecting our health or limiting our potential.

Good luck on your journey!

Notes

Chapter 2
1. See, for example, the Concise Oxford English Dictionary, which among other things defines stress as 'a state of mental, emotional or other strain'.

2. This is the system affected by most anti-depressants, including Prozac.

Chapter 3
1. Thomas H. Holmes and Richard H. Rahe, 'The Social Readjustment Rating Scale', *Journal of Psychosomatic Research*, volume 1, issue 2, 1967, pages 213–18.

Chapter 4
1. Pre-eclampsia is a serious condition, usually detected when blood pressure starts to rise during pregnancy. It can carry serious risks for both mother and child, and can mean that a baby needs to be delivered early.

2. For a much more detailed account of the many impacts of stress, I'd recommend: Robert M. Sapolsky, *Why Zebras Don't Get Ulcers: The Acclaimed Guide to Stress, Stress-related Diseases, and Coping*, St Martin's Press Inc., 2004.

Chapter 7
1. To use his words, 'the bodily changes follow directly the perception of the exciting fact... our feeling of the same changes as they occur *is* the emotion'. William James, *What is an Emotion?*, 1884, page 247.

2. Antonio Damasio. *Descartes' Error: Emotion, Reason and the Human Brain*, Vintage, 2006, page 115.

Chapter 10
1. Of these, the best-known free websites are MoodGym – http://moodgym.anu.edu.au/welcome – and Living Life to the Full – http://www.livinglifetothefull.com. Both require you to register but then take you through a course of CBT, week by week.

Chapter 11
1. Published by Robinson, 1999.

Chapter 13
1. If you're interested in the figures, studies suggest that drinking one large glass of wine each night (which can easily be as much as three units) raises the risk of breast cancer by one fifth. Drinking two large glasses raises it by one third and drinking three large glasses results in an increase of more than 50 per cent.

Chapter 14
1. Chronic pain triggers the release of the same hormones that are involved in chronic stress, so if you have a condition causing you a lot of pain, it will make you more prone to problems with stress. Ask your doctor for help with pain management or a referral to a pain clinic for more support.

Chapter 17
1. If you're in this position, spare a thought for the family of former US president Theodore Roosevelt, whose snoring was apparently so bad that when he stayed in a hotel, all the

other guests on his floor had to be relocated so that he didn't keep them awake.

2. This is also why jet lag can be such a problem. Quite simply, our body's clock is out of sync with the actual time in the place we have just got to, and this takes time to adjust. Luckily your clock does reset with exposure to daylight, so try to spend the days in natural daylight when you can and the nights in the dark or in dimmed light. Hopefully you'll soon be back on schedule – usually just in time to go home again!